Veterinary Ophthalmology: a manual for nurses and technicians

C000048620

For Elsevier:

Commissioning Editor: Mary Seager
Development Editor: Rebecca Nelemans
Project Manager: David Fleming
Designer: Andy Chapman
Illustration Manager: Bruce Hogarth

Veterinary Ophthalmology

A manual for nurses and technicians

Sally Turner MA VetMB DVOphthal MRCVS
RCVS Specialist in Veterinary Ophthalmology

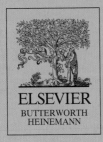

ELSEVIER
BUTTERWORTH
HEINEMANN

Edinburgh   London   New York   Oxford   Philadelphia   St Louis   Sydney   Toronto   2005

ELSEVIER
BUTTERWORTH
HEINEMANN

© 2005, Elsevier Limited. All rights reserved.

No part of this publication may be reproduced, stored in a retrieval system, or transmitted in any form or by any means, electronic, mechanical, photocopying, recording or otherwise, without either the prior permission of the publishers or a licence permitting restricted copying in the United Kingdom issued by the Copyright Licensing Agency, 90 Tottenham Court Road, London W1T 4LP. Permissions may be sought directly from Elsevier's Health Sciences Rights Department in Philadelphia, USA: phone: (+1) 215 238 7869, fax: (+1) 215 238 2239, e-mail: healthpermissions@elsevier.com. You may also complete your request on-line via the Elsevier homepage (http://www.elsevier.com), by selecting 'Customer Support' and then 'Obtaining Permissions'.

First published 2005

ISBN 0 7506 8841 6

British Library Cataloguing in Publication Data
A catalogue record for this book is available from the British Library

Library of Congress Cataloging in Publication Data
A catalog record for this book is available from the Library of Congress

Knowledge and best practice in this field are constantly changing. As new research and experience broaden our knowledge, changes in practice, treatment and drug therapy may become necessary or appropriate. Readers are advised to check the most current information provided (i) on procedures featured or (ii) by the manufacturer of each product to be administered, to verify the recommended dose or formula, the method and duration of administration, and contraindications. It is the responsibility of the practitioner, relying on their own experience and knowledge of the patient, to make diagnoses, to determine dosages and the best treatment for each individual patient, and to take all appropriate safety precautions. To the fullest extent of the law, neither the publisher nor the author assumes any liability for any injury and/or damage.

The Publisher

The publisher's policy is to use **paper manufactured from sustainable forests**

Printed in China

Contents

To Jeff, for his love and support, and to Jean and Trevor, for providing the genes!

Preface

As veterinary medicine has undergone a transformation in the last decade, with more emphasis on specialisation and a proliferation of private referral centres, so the need for the speciality nurse is increasing. Hence, the need for a book such as this. Ophthalmology is an area which is often covered in minimal detail in general nursing training, and because it includes both medical and surgical conditions, it is not fully addressed in courses which specialise in either of these disciplines—the most frequently encountered post-qualification areas of specialisation available to nurses. As such, many nurses, even those with a lot of experience, still feel overwhelmed by ophthalmology—the eyes are such delicate and emotive structures, the terminology involved with ocular disease is another language altogether and the challenge of successful treatments can make the management of the patient with ocular disease a daunting prospect. I hope that this book will provide a user-friendly text which will both inform and educate, while at the same time inspire its readers to understand what a wonderful subject ophthalmology is!

This book is intended for all nurses and technicians who are interested in veterinary ophthalmology. It provides a hands-on approach which will be of value to student nurses, those in general practice as well as those in speciality ophthalmic referral centres. In addition, it will be useful for veterinary students wishing to gain a basic understanding of this fascinating discipline, as well as general practitioners looking for a concise text for easy reference. It is designed to provide useful, practical advice for nursing the patient with ocular disease, with special emphasis on dogs and cats (although sections on horses, rabbits and other small animals are included).

The book starts with a short chapter on anatomy and physiology—essential for gaining a basic understanding of the structure of the eye and how it works. A section is included here on vision in animals. A chapter on ocular pharmacology and therapeutics follows, with detailed instructions on how to apply different ocular medications—the emphasis is on practicality rather than an exhaustive list of possible treatments. The chapter on the ophthalmic examination is comprehensive and includes all the ancillary tests which might be required in reaching a diagnosis—many of these tests can be undertaken by nurses, while their assistance with the examination itself is invaluable. Special chapters on medical and surgical nursing then follow, the latter including surgical equipment and instruments found in ophthalmic practice. Since there are many special factors to consider with anaesthesia of patients for ocular surgery, a separate chapter is dedicated to this subject. Two clinical chapters, on general and specialised ophthalmic conditions and procedures come next. Here details of the ocular conditions are discussed with special emphasis on the role of the nurse for each disease mentioned. A short chapter is included on canine inherited eye disease. A comprehensive glossary is included since ophthalmic terminology is often complicated and can be confusing! For quick reference, there are three appendices: the first provides a summary of ophthalmic emergencies, the second covers causes of blindness, and the third lists suppliers for ophthalmology instruments, equipment and disposable items.

The book is abundantly illustrated throughout with clear, easily understood line diagrams, together with numerous colour photographs. These are essential to the understanding of ophthalmic problems—it is, after all, a very visual subject!

Acknowledgements

I would like to thank the veterinary surgeons who have referred cases to me—photographs of some of these are scattered throughout the book. I also acknowledge all the nurses I have worked with over the years *(you know who you are!)*—many of you have inspired me during the writing of this text! I am very grateful to Gerard Brouwer for his advice and comments on the anaesthesia chapter—much appreciated! I would like to thank Dennis Brooks for the loan of some equine slides (acknowledged individually) and Tony Read for providing me with information on Australian suppliers.

1 Anatomy and physiology

INTRODUCTION

A good understanding of basic ocular anatomy and the physiological functions of the various structures involved is essential before disease processes and ophthalmic nursing can be considered. The eye is a unique sensory organ which allows awareness of the surroundings by the processing of light into electrical signals that are interpreted in the brain. The basic structure of the mammalian eye is similar in all species, but various adaptations have developed to enhance the evolutionary role of the species concerned. For example, dogs and cats are mainly nocturnal and their eyes have adapted to have improved night vision. Horses and other herbivores have widely spaced eyes on the side of their heads to extend their visual fields such that they can see potential predators without needing to move their heads. We will consider some of these adaptations later in this chapter.

ORBIT

The orbit is the bony fossa which separates the eye from the cranial cavity. It surrounds and protects the globe while providing a route for vessels and nerves to access the eye. In addition to the eye itself, this region contains the extraocular muscles, optic nerve and lacrimal gland, along with blood vessels and nerves (Fig. 1.1). In man, the bony surround is complete, providing excellent protection to the globe from all directions. However, in carnivores there are areas where only soft tissue surrounds the eye. These areas are mainly ventral to the globe, where the masseter and pterygoid muscles provide the floor of the orbit, and are of relevance when considering retrobulbar disease. Conditions involving these muscles of mastication, as well as those in the caudal molars, caudal nasal chambers and zygomatic salivary glands, can all affect the eye due to the close anatomic connection. Thus, a dog presenting with a retrobulbar problem needs to have a careful oral examination—a tooth root abscess affecting a molar tooth could easily be contributing to the ocular signs. Disease processes affecting

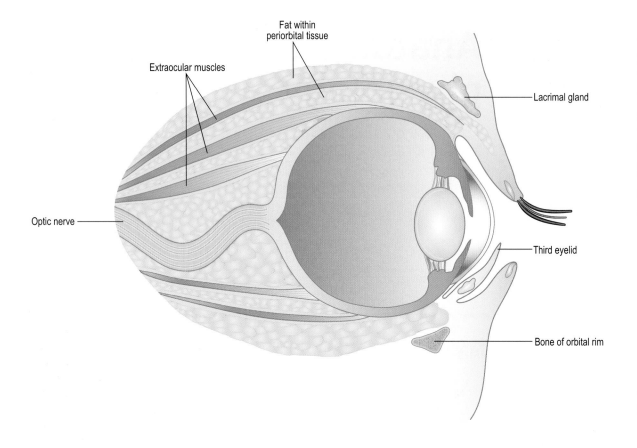

Fat within
periorbital tissue

Extraocular muscles

Lacrimal gland

Optic nerve

Third eyelid

Bone of orbital rim

Fig. 1.1 Contents of the orbit.

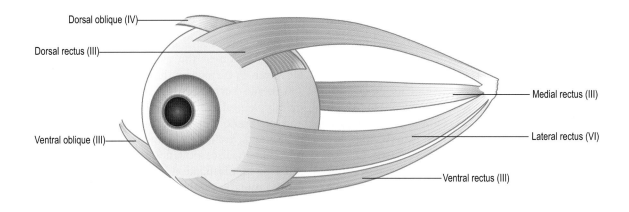

Dorsal oblique (IV)

Dorsal rectus (III)

Medial rectus (III)

Lateral rectus (VI)

Ventral oblique (III)

Ventral rectus (III)

Fig. 1.2 The extraocular muscles and their innervation.

the frontal and maxillary sinuses can also lead to ocular involvement by local spread of infectious, inflammatory or neoplastic conditions.

The extraocular muscles are located within the orbit. They are normal striated muscle and are attached to the globe to provide ocular motility. There are six muscles for each eye (Fig. 1.2): the four rectus muscles (dorsal, ventral, medial and lateral; pull the eye in their respective directions), the dorsal oblique (which pulls the dorsolateral aspect of the globe ventromedially) and the ventral oblique (which pulls the eye mediodorsally). The extraocular muscles are innervated by the oculomotor nerve (cranial nerve III), apart from the lateral rectus muscle which is innervated by the abducens nerve (cranial nerve VI) and the dorsal oblique muscle which is supplied by the trochlear nerve (cranial nerve IV). Thus, if there are abnormalities with the cranial nerves this can affect both the position of the eye within the socket and its movement. These findings can aid with the localisation of any lesion and form an important part of neuro-ophthalmology. In addition to the muscles, orbital fat fills the space around the eye within the orbit. This allows the eye to move within the socket when pulled by the extraocular muscles, and also provides protective cushioning (e.g. in blunt trauma).

EYELIDS

The eyelids are dorsal and ventral folds of skin lined with palpebral conjunctiva. Within these folds are various structures. A fibrous layer, called the tarsal plate, provides support. This is less well developed in dogs than cats. In addition to providing support, the eyelid folds also contain both smooth and striated muscles (the latter include the orbicularis oculi muscles), and a good vascular and nerve supply (Fig. 1.3). The eyelids meet at the lateral and medial canthus, and the opening formed by their free edges is called the palpebral fissure (Fig. 1.4). Palpebral ligaments are present

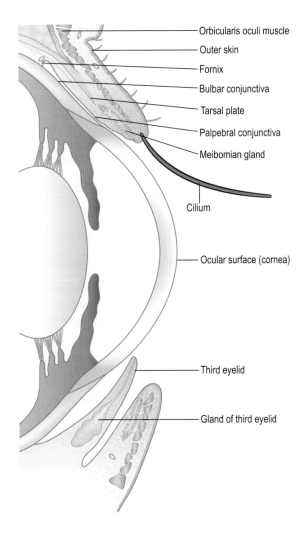

- Orbicularis oculi muscle
- Outer skin
- Fornix
- Bulbar conjunctiva
- Tarsal plate
- Palpebral conjunctiva
- Meibomian gland
- Cilium
- Ocular surface (cornea)
- Third eyelid
- Gland of third eyelid

Fig. 1.3 Anatomy of the canine eyelids.

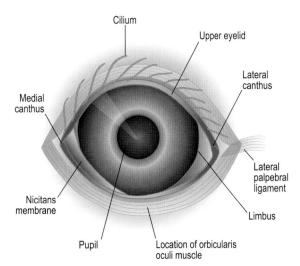

Cilium
Upper eyelid
Lateral canthus
Medial canthus
Lateral palpebral ligament
Nicitans membrane
Limbus
Pupil
Location of orbicularis oculi muscle

Fig. 1.4 Appearance of the canine eye showing adnexal structures.

medially and laterally, and these fibrous bands stabilise the lids and help to maintain the shape of the palpebral fissure. Eyelid sensation is provided by the trigeminal nerve (cranial nerve V). The lids are closed by contraction of the orbicularis oculi muscle, which is innervated by the facial nerve (cranial nerve VII). The rapid action of this muscle is important for globe protection and in the distribution of the tear film. The normal position of the eyelids is resting against the ocular surface, and they slide over it during blinking. Many breeds of dogs and cats have poor lid–globe apposition, and this results in ocular problems such as entropion (rolling-in of the eyelids) or ectropion (rolling-out of the eyelids). These conditions are discussed in Chapter 7.

Along the free margin of the lids (especially the upper lid) are a row of cilia (not true eyelashes). These are located close to, but not actually on, the eyelid margin. Within the eyelid margins are meibomian glands (also called tarsal glands), which secrete the oily (lipid) portion of the tear film. These are shown in Figure 1.3. The eyelid margin itself is normally totally free from hairs and can be pigmented. The eyelid skin is very thin and easily becomes inflamed and oedematous (numerous mast cells within it contribute to this)—thus many clinical problems can occur in this area.

The third eyelid or nictitating membrane (membrana nictitans) is a ventromedial fold of conjunctiva containing a T-shaped cartilage for support with the nictitans gland at its base (which together with the lacrimal gland produces the aqueous portion of the tear film). The leading edge of the third eyelid is often pigmented. However, in some dogs, particularly those with parti-coloured coats, one eye might have a pigmented border while the other is non-pigmented. This is a completely normal variation and should not be confused with inflammation (the pink third eyelid is more noticeable against the darker colour of the iris than the pigmented one and owners often think that the dog has conjunctivitis in one eye). The third eyelid sweeps across the globe during blinking and assists in spreading the tear film and removing debris. It can be likened to a windscreen wiper in this respect. Unlike dogs, cats have some striated muscle fibres present within their third eyelids, which allow for active protrusion of the membrane.

CONJUNCTIVA

The conjunctiva is the thin mucous membrane which lines the eyelids and the exposed portion of sclera. It is divided into three sections:
- palpebral (lining the lids)
- bulbar (overlying the globe)
- nictitans (covering the third eyelid).

The palpebral conjunctiva starts at the eyelid margin and lines both upper and lower lids. It meets the bulbar conjunctiva at the fornix where the conjunctiva is reflected over the sclera of the globe (Fig. 1.3). The bulbar conjunctiva continues to the limbus. The conjunctiva contains goblet cells in its outer epithelium (which produce the mucoid portion of the tear film), lymphoid tissue in its middle layer, and connective tissue, blood vessels and nerves in the deepest layer. The bright red branching blood vessels can be easily seen, especially in the bulbar conjunctiva. Sensory nerves are branches of the trigeminal nerve (cranial nerve V). Variable amounts of pigment are also present. The conjunctiva is freely mobile except at the limbus and eyelid margins. Functions of the conjunctiva include preventing corneal desiccation, increasing eyelid mobility and providing a barrier to microorganisms and foreign bodies.

THE LACRIMAL SYSTEM

The lacrimal system is made up of a secretory component (pre-ocular tear film) and an excretory component (nasolacrimal drainage system).

Pre-ocular tear film

An adequate supply of tears is necessary to maintain ocular integrity and normal function. The pre-ocular tear film covers the corneal and conjunctival surfaces, and its close proximity to these underlying structures means that it is important in both health and disease. The pre-ocular tear film has a pH of 6.8–8.0 (mean 7.5). This is important when considering topical medication; for example, drops with a different pH are more likely to sting on application. Functions of the pre-ocular tear film include the following:

- maintaining an optically uniform corneal surface
- removing foreign material and debris from the conjunctiva and cornea
- permitting the passage of oxygen and nutrients
- possessing anti-bacterial properties.

Traditionally the pre-ocular tear film is considered to be made up of three layers, although the structure and interactions of these layers is probably much more complicated than this! These layers are:

1. *Outer oily layer.* This thin layer is produced by the meibomian glands. The glands are present in the palpebral conjunctiva with their openings visible as a line of grey dots on the eyelid margin. This layer helps to decrease evaporation, improves the stability of the whole of the tear film and provides a protective oily barrier at the lid margins.

2. *Middle aqueous layer.* This is produced from lacrimal and third eyelid glands and constitutes the bulk of the tear film. The lacrimal gland, located dorsolateral to the globe within the periorbita of the lacrimal bone, provides the majority of the aqueous tear production with the nictitans gland producing approximately $\frac{1}{4}$ to $\frac{1}{3}$ of the total amount. This aqueous layer allows oxygen and nutrient diffusion and facilitates smooth movement of the eyeball, as well as contributing to corneal protection.

3. *Inner mucin layer.* This thin layer is produced by conjunctival goblet cells. It adheres to the cornea, allowing the aqueous layer to spread easily and evenly over the surface.

Blinking spreads the tear film, and the blink rate is increased with pain or ocular discomfort (blepharospasm). An increased blink rate is also seen in restrained animals, which is one reason why it is important to watch the animal prior to handling in order to accurately assess blinking.

Nasolacrimal drainage

The tear film is continually produced in the normal eye and, therefore, needs to be drained away as well (only a small amount is lost by evaporation). The tears drain down the nasolacrimal duct through the upper and lower nasolacrimal punctae close to the medial canthus (Fig. 1.5). It is of note

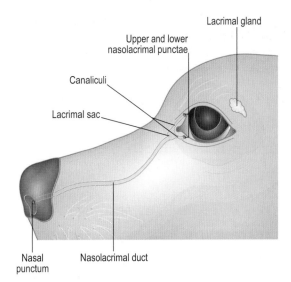

Fig. 1.5 Nasolacrimal drainage system.

that rabbits only have a lower punctum. Tears drain to the nasal cavity and the back of the mouth (patency can be checked by instilling fluorescein dye into the conjunctival sac and watching it appear at the nostril or in the mouth, or by cannulating and flushing the system). During blinking, tears are thought to be propelled medially and into the punctae and, as such, the process is active as well as passive due to gravity. Anatomical problems in this area frequently lead to tear overflow or epiphora. For example, a small (micropunctum) or absent (imperforate) ventral nasolacrimal punctum will not allow proper tear drainage, nor will poor lid apposition in this area.

THE GLOBE

The eyeball itself is made up of three layers (Table 1.1). Figure 1.6 shows a cross section through the eye. Most of the internal structures of the eye are transparent: the aqueous and vitreous humours and the lens. They refract (bend the angle of) and transmit light to the retina and provide internal pressure to keep the globe normally distended.

The cornea

The cornea is the clear, avascular anterior portion of the fibrous coating of the globe. It is less than

Table 1.1 The layers of the globe

Layer	Name	Function
Outer	Cornea and sclera	Provides support and maintains shape Anterior portion clear to assist passage of light
Middle	Uvea (choroid, ciliary body and iris)	Provides nutrition, modifies light entering eye via pupil
Inner	Retina and optic nerve	Conversion of light impulses to electrical signals for central processing

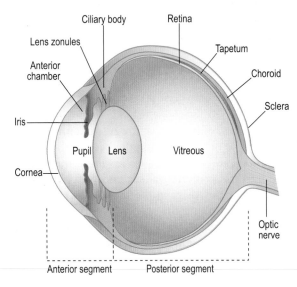

Fig. 1.6 Cross section of the eye showing internal structures.

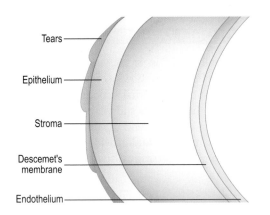

Fig. 1.7 Cross section of the cornea showing its different layers. (From Grahn 2004, with permission of Butterworth Heinemann)

0.7 mm thick in dogs and cats. It is made up of an outer epithelium, middle stroma and inner endothelium (Fig. 1.7). A very thin, elastic layer (Descemet's membrane) separates the stroma from the endothelium. The epithelium consists of several layers of cells attached to a basement membrane. The stroma is the thickest layer, made up of special corneal cells called keratocytes and regularly arranged collagen fibrils with a ground substance (which helps with the nutrition of the layer; there are no blood vessels to provide this). The corneal stroma is richly supplied with sensory nerves (trigeminal, cranial nerve V), which branch superficially (hence shallow corneal ulcers are more painful than deeper ones). The endothelium is composed of a single layer of cells with little capacity for regeneration during life.

Corneal transparency is maintained by:

- lack of blood vessels
- non-keratinised surface epithelium
- lack of pigment
- size and organisation of collagen fibres within the stroma.

Any alteration in these factors will cause some opacification of the cornea which, if severe, will have a deleterious affect on vision.

The sclera

The sclera is the thick, fibrous outer layer of the posterior globe. It merges with the cornea at the limbus, which forms the transition zone between these two structures and is a 1 mm wide, variably pigmented band. It contains a population of corneal stem cells which are important during corneal wound healing. The sclera itself is a much larger structure than the cornea and is composed of collagen fibres which are thicker and less regular than in the cornea. It also contains some elastic fibres and a modest number of blood vessels and sensory nerves. The sclera usually appears white in colour, but if the sclera is thinned for any reason, the dark underlying choroid can be partially visible rendering the sclera pale blue in colour. The episclera overlies the sclera and is a thin fibroelastic structure which is highly vascular.

The uveal tract

The uveal tract makes up the middle layer of the globe and consists of the iris, ciliary body and choroid. It is usually pigmented.

Iris

The iris is the visible, coloured layer seen within the eye. It consists of an anterior layer of stroma and iris sphincter muscle, and a posterior layer made up of an epithelial layer (which is pigmented) and dilator muscle. The colour of the iris depends on both the number of pigment cells (melanocytes) present in the stroma and the thickness of the anterior layer itself. The hole in the centre of the iris is the pupil. Movement of the iris muscles controls the quantity of light entering the posterior segment through the pupil. The sphincter muscle circles the pupil in the dog, while in the cat the fibres also criss-cross above and below the pupil, allowing it to constrict to a narrow vertical slit. Other species such as horses, sheep and reptiles have different arrangements of this muscle which contribute to pupil shape. Constriction of the pupil is mediated via parasympathetic nerve fibres travelling in the oculomotor nerve (cranial nerve III). The dilator muscle is innervated by sympathetic fibres which run with the ophthalmic branch of the trigeminal nerve (cranial nerve V). The dilator muscle radiates out from the pupil margin towards the iris periphery in a similar pattern to bicycle spokes. In addition to regulating the amount of light entering, altering pupil size also affects depth of focus and reduces optical aberrations.

Ciliary body

The ciliary body is located behind the iris, between the lens and choroid (Fig. 1.6). It can be divided into sections containing the ciliary processes and the ciliary body musculature. It also forms part of the iridocorneal angle (ICA). The ciliary processes secrete aqueous humour; the transparent fluid which fills the anterior and posterior chambers. Aqueous provides nutrients to, and removes waste products from, the avascular structures within the anterior part of the eye (i.e. the lens and cornea). Aqueous drains from the eye mainly through the iridocorneal angle (Fig. 1.8). Pectinate ligaments span the opening to the ICA (see Fig. 3.17, p. 41). The balance between production and outflow of aqueous creates the intraocular pressure; imbalance can lead to raised intraocular pressure (glaucoma) or lowered pressure (hypotony). The ciliary body epithelium forms part of the 'blood–aqueous barrier', protecting ocular metabolism. Breakdown of this barrier occurs with inflammation, trauma, surgery and some drugs, and results in leakage of proteins and other blood-borne components into the aqueous. In addition to its metabolic functions, the ciliary body provides attachments for the lens (via the lens zonules) and has some effect on accommo-

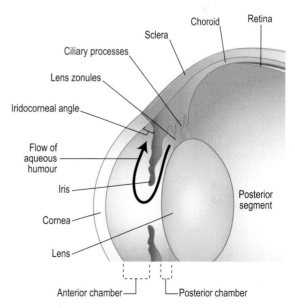

Fig. 1.8 The production and drainage of aqueous humour.

dation (focussing). However, this process is poorly developed in animals and the ciliary muscle does not alter the shape of the lens for focussing in the same way as it does in people (see 'Vision in dogs and cats', p. 10).

Choroid

The choroid is the posterior portion of the uveal tract and lies between the sclera and retina. It is made up of several layers and contains many thin-walled blood vessels and pigmented support tissues. Within the dorsal portion of the choroid is found the tapetum lucidum, or simply the tapetum. This is a mirror-like layer (responsible for the eye shine seen in dogs and cats) which functions to re-stimulate the retinal photoreceptors when light is reflected back from it. This increases visual sensitivity and assists vision in low light intensity. The choroid also provides glucose and oxygen for retinal metabolism.

The lens

The lens is a transparent bi-concave structure encased in a capsule (Fig. 1.9). At its periphery

(equator), lens zonules attach it to the ciliary processes. The iris rests on its anterior surface and glides over it as the pupil opens and closes. The adult lens contains no blood vessels or pigment, which would reduce its transparency. Any opacity in the lens or its capsule is termed a cataract. Lens fibres make up the bulk of the structure, and a Y shape (called a suture line) is formed both anteriorly and posteriorly where the ends of the fibres meet. The anterior Y suture is the right way up while the posterior suture is inverted (like a Mercedes sign). This fact is helpful when identifying the position of cataracts within the lens. The central portion of the lens is called the nucleus, and is the first part of the lens to form during embryogenesis. Hardening of this central portion is seen in older animals and gives a blue-grey appearance to the lens. This can be mistaken for a cataract, but nuclear sclerosis, as it is termed, does not affect vision significantly. Surrounding the nucleus is the cortex of the lens. Beneath the anterior lens capsule lies the lens epithelium, which secretes new lens fibres during life. This is the only part of the normal lens which is metabolically active. The lens in animals is proportionally larger than in man, i.e. it takes up a greater volume compared to the rest of the globe. As mentioned above, changes in muscle tone of the ciliary body musculature alter the shape (and thus optical power) of the lens in man, a process called accommodation. This is very limited in dogs and cats. The nutritional and oxygen requirements of the lens are supplied by the aqueous.

The vitreous

The vitreous is the largest single structure of the eye and forms $2/3$ the volume of the globe. It fills the posterior segment of the globe between the back of the lens, ciliary body and retina. It is a transparent jelly-like substance (hydro-gel) which transmits light, maintains the shape of the eyeball, provides cushioning during eye movements and keeps the retina in its normal position.

The retina

The retina is a very complex structure, which is similar in conformation to the brain. It forms the

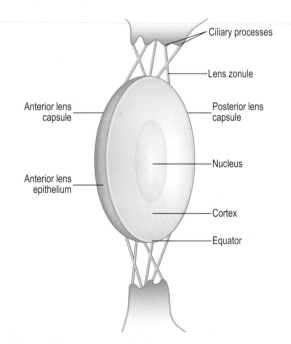

Anterior lens capsule

Anterior lens epithelium

Ciliary processes

Lens zonule

Posterior lens capsule

Nucleus

Cortex

Equator

Fig. 1.9 The anatomy of the lens.

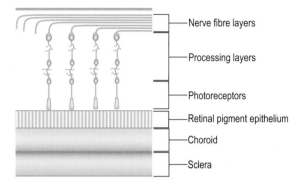

Nerve fibre layers

Processing layers

Photoreceptors

Retinal pigment epithelium

Choroid

Sclera

Fig. 1.10 Simplified schematic diagram of the retina.

inner-most layer of the back of the globe and comprises ten separate layers which can be distinguished histologically, and are simplified in Figure 1.10. The innermost of these layers (closest to the vitreous) is the nerve fibre layer. The nerve fibres converge at the optic disc and exit the globe as the optic nerve (cranial nerve II). Several layers of transmitting cells are present beneath the nerve fibre layer, and on the outside of these is the photoreceptor layer. The photoreceptors are specialised cells which contain photopigments that alter on exposure to light. This chemical energy is changed to electrical energy, which is transmitted as impulses to the visual cortex in the brain and interpreted as vision. Two types of photoreceptors are present:

● *Rods* function best in dim light and are present in much greater numbers.
● *Cones* are adapted for bright light conditions, sharp acuity and have some colour detection in dogs and cats (less well-developed than in man).

Cone concentration is highest centrally (around the area centralis, dorsolateral to the optic disc). The outermost layer of the retina is the retinal pigment epithelium (RPE) which lies adjacent to the choroid. It provides metabolites for the photoreceptors and removes their waste products (the rest of the retina receives nutrients from the choroidal capillaries or via diffusion from the vitreous). As its name suggests, the RPE is normally pigmented (with melanin). However, it contains no melanin in the area which has the tapetum within the choroid beneath it. This allows light to be transmitted through the RPE to the tapetum,

which reflects it back onto the photoreceptors a second time. This process improves visual perception in low light levels.

The optic nerve and central visual pathways

The nerve fibre layer of the retina converges at the optic disc to form the optic nerve (cranial nerve II). This passes out from the back of the eye through the retrobulbar tissues and into the skull. The two optic nerves meet at the optic chiasm, where some crossing over of nerve fibres occurs. The optic tracts then continue into the brain and up to the visual cortex. Complex interactions occur within the brain which contribute to visual awareness, pupillary light reflexes, blinking and various other neuro-ophthalmological reactions.

EMBRYOLOGY OF THE EYE

An understanding of basic embryology is helpful since it allows us to relate the different structures of the eye to each other, as well as making sense of some congenital ocular abnormalities (which can occur particularly in pedigree animals). Unfortunately, the development of the eye is extremely complex! The eye starts to form early in gestation and develops as an outpocket of the early forebrain, the optic vesicle. It remains attached to the forebrain by the optic stalk and grows outwards to contact the surface of the developing foetus (surface ectoderm) where the lens starts to develop. The optic vesicle envelops the forming lens but does not fully enclose it; the future cornea also forms from the surface rather than the optic vesicle (Fig. 1.11). Within the vesicle, the layers start to differentiate into the uveal tract, retina and so on. The growing structure gains nutrition and oxygen supplies from the hyaloid vessels, which enter through the ventral aspect of the vesicle. Sometimes remnants of these embryonic vessels can be found as persistent pupillary membrane remnants or persistent hyperplastic primary vitreous (see Chapter 7 for more information). Failure of normal embryogenesis can also lead to a small eye (microphthalmos), colobomas (holes or absence of tissue where certain parts of the vesicle fail to

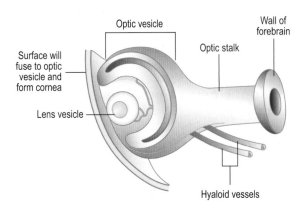

Surface will
fuse to optic
vesicle and
form cornea

Optic vesicle

Optic stalk

Wall of
forebrain

Lens vesicle

Hyaloid vessels

Fig. 1.11 Schematic diagram of the developing eye.

fuse normally), retinal dysplasia (where the retinal layers do not form properly) and multiple ocular abnormalities.

VISION IN DOGS AND CATS

Do dogs and cats see the world in the same way as us? This is a question that interests many people (whether they own animals or not). The simple answer is 'no they do not', but since vision is such a subjective thing it is not easy to say exactly how other animals see. It is necessary to bear in mind several different visual parameters and address each in turn when considering the differences and similarities between our visual awareness and that of our pets. Areas to address include vision in differing light intensities, visual acuity, movement and depth perception and ability to detect different colours and shapes.

Vision in differing light intensities

Dogs and cats have a greater visual ability in low light conditions than humans (i.e. they see better than we do in the dark), yet they also still retain good visual function in a wide range of lighting levels, including daylight. Thus, their visual system is not highly adapted for either nocturnal or strictly diurnal vision. The minimal threshold of light for vision in cats is about 6 times lower than man, and it is similar for dogs. This makes investigation of their responses in low level illumination difficult, since human experimenters cannot use

their own senses to record the animal's response! In dogs, the central area of the retina predominantly consists of rod photoreceptors, which are sensitive to low light intensities. In man this same area of retina is mainly populated by cone photoreceptors. In addition, there are different sensitivities of the rod photopigment, rhodopsin, between man and dog.

In most dogs and cats there is also the presence of the mirror-like tapetum lucidum in the dorsal fundus. This is thought to reflect light back through the photoreceptors a second time, thus optimising each ray of light. In fact, the feline tapetum is thought to reflect 130 times more light than does the human eye (at a price though, since this reflection leads to scattering of light which may reduce acuity). The tapetum is also thought to subtly shift the wavelengths of the reflected light via fluorescence, which results in greater enhancement of contrast.

Motion perception

The perception of motion is critically important for dogs and cats, and they are able to detect smaller movements at a greater distance away than humans can. They also have a greater sensitivity to flickering lights than do people. In humans, the point at which a flickering light appears to fuse to a constantly illuminated light (flicker fusion) is about 50–60 Hz for cone (daylight) receptors. Dogs have a flicker fusion of about 70–80 Hz in similar lighting conditions. This means that to us a television screen appears as a fluidly moving story, with the screen updated at 60 times a second, while to most dogs it would appear to flicker rapidly.

Visual perspective

Another point to consider is visual perspective. When standing, we see the world from a height of about 1.5 metres or more above the ground. Compare this to a cat or small dog at a few centimetres, a Labrador at 50 cm and an Irish wolfhound at a metre. Certainly their perspectives would be different.

Depth perception

Depth perception is directly related to the visual field and degree of binocular overlap, where the two eyes view the same scene from slightly differing positions. The brain then compares the two images and creates a three-dimensional image (stereopsis). In cats, the eyes are directed fairly forwards giving a large angle of binocular overlap while in some canine breeds they are more lateral. The presence of a long nose can reduce binocular overlap, while enucleation removes it completely! One-eyed dogs and cats adapt very quickly to monocular vision and rarely seem to have difficulties in judging distances and so on. In this instance, monocular clues, including brightness, contour, shadows, aerial perspective, object overlay and parallax, are used as markers.

Visual acuity

Visual acuity refers to the ability to see the details of an object separately and unblurred. It depends on the optical properties of the eye, the retina and the ability of the higher visual pathways to interpret the images. It is also affected by lighting levels, with cone acuity far higher than when the rods alone are stimulated in dim light. Optical properties of the eye are the first factors to consider. The rays of light pass through the cornea, aqueous humour, lens, vitreous and then form a focussed image on the retina. Clearly, myopia (short-sightedness) or hypermetropia (long-sight-

edness) will result in an out-of-focus image on the retina and, thus, reduced acuity. Mild myopia is reported in some breeds (e.g. German shepherd dogs and rottweilers), but functionally does not seem to be a problem in the canine population. Astigmatism, where the corneal curvature is not symmetrical, is also relatively uncommon in dogs and cats, but can be induced pathologically. Corneal disease, focal cataracts or adhesions (synechia) can all affect the transmission of parallel rays of light through the optical system.

The ability to focus on objects at differing distances from the retina is called accommodation. In humans this occurs mainly through contraction and relaxation of the ciliary muscles, leading to increased and decreased refractive power of the lens and focusing of close and distant objects, respectively. In dogs and cats, lens elasticity is minimal and focusing is achieved by movements in the position of the whole lens (translation). Their ability to accommodate is much lower than ours (2–3 dioptres in dogs versus 14 dioptres in children) and close objects always remain blurred. Pupil size also affects visual acuity, since a smaller pupil has a greater depth of focus but allows less light to pass through. The pupillary light reflex is a constant balance between maximal illumination and maximal resolution.

Retinal factors affecting visual acuity include the density of rod and cone photoreceptors in different areas of the retina, the presence of a fovea (man) or an area centralis (dogs and cats) and the numbers of optic nerve fibres.

Colour perception

Colour perception is an interesting topic, as owners always want to know if their pets can see in colour. Most people are trichromatic (i.e. they see in three colours: red, blue and green, which then mix to create the full colour spectrum). Dogs and cats are dichromatic, and lack green-sensitive cones. Their vision is thought to be similar to a human who is red-green colour blind. This means that they see blue and yellow well but have trouble with reds and greens: red appears dark, and green is indistinguishable from white. Thus, a cat sees a green lawn as a whitish lawn, and a green rosebush with red flowers as a whitish bush with dark flowers. This is assuming that the cat actually perceives the wavelengths of light as colour in the same way as we do—and this is a major assumption! The guide dog for a blind person at the traffic lights will be responding to the brightness and position of the lights and not their colour! In addition, we must remember that dogs and cats have very few cones in their central retina: probably less than 10% compared to 100% cones in the same area of retina in a human. Thus, perception of colour must be much poorer than in people.

In summary we can conclude that the visual system of dogs and cats is different from ours. Their eyes function better in poor light, have a wider field of view and an enhanced ability to detect motion. However, colour perception, accommodative ability and visual acuity are superior in humans.

BIBLIOGRAPHY AND FURTHER READING

Gelatt KN. Veterinary ophthalmology. 3rd edn. Philadelphia: Lippincott Williams & Wilkins; 1999.

Grahn B, Cullen C, Peiffer R. Veterinary ophthalmology essentials. Oxford: Butterworth-Heinemann; 2004.

Slatter D. Fundamentals of veterinary ophthalmology. 3rd edn. London: WB Saunders; 2001.

2 Ocular pharmacology and therapeutics

INTRODUCTION

The aim of ocular therapy is to reach sufficiently high drug concentrations in the target tissues without building up toxic concentrations in other ocular tissues or elsewhere in the body. The eye is a very delicate yet highly complex structure, and the successful management of ocular disease depends not only on an accurate diagnosis by the veterinary surgeon, but also an understanding of ocular pharmacology, such that the most appropriate medications are chosen and applied in the most effective manner. The eyes are designed to be protected from external stimuli, and anatomical features (such as the structure of the cornea) and shielding mechanisms (such as the tear film) can act as barriers to effective topical treatment. Therefore, when medicating eyes we need to remember where we want the drug to go and in what concentration, and this will affect our choice of route and frequency of administration.

We can think of the eye as composed of several compartments separated by semi-permeable barriers. The drug barriers of the eye are the cornea, the blood–aqueous barrier and the blood–retinal barrier (the latter two make up the blood–ocular barrier). Areas which might require medication can be divided into the following:

- extraocular structures
- iris tissue
- ciliary body
- vitreous and retina
- retrobulbar structures.

These are detailed further in Table 2.1.

Another factor to consider when choosing a route for medication is owner compliance. It is vital to show owners how to apply topical medications: asking if they know how to apply them is not sufficient. Ideally, you should show the owner how to medicate one eye and then get them to demonstrate their proficiency on the other one (see below for details of how to apply topical medication, and Chapter 4). In addition to being capable

Table 2.1 Ocular targets for drug therapy

Site	Tissues involved	Examples of drug type
Adnexal and surface structures	Eyelids Conjunctiva Cornea	Antimicrobial agents Anti-inflammatory agents
Iris	Dilator or constrictor muscles	Mydriatic agents (pupil-dilating) Miotics (pupil-constricting)
Ciliary body	Aqueous-producing epithelial cells	Ocular hypotensive agents in glaucoma treatment
Posterior segment	Vitreous Choroid Retina	Immunosuppressive agents for panuveitis Antimicrobials
Retrobulbar tissue	Muscles, nerves and connective tissue	Anaesthetic agents in retrobulbar anaesthesia Antimicrobial agents

of administering the treatment, the owner must have the time to treat the patient for the specified period and should be aware of what to expect in terms of improvement or deterioration of the condition. It is pointless suggesting 6× daily medication if the owner is out at work all day with no one to help with treating. In these instances, a longer-acting preparation or alternative route of administration might be appropriate.

ROUTES OF ADMINISTRATION

Various routes of administration are possible when treating ocular diseases. These include topical, local injections and systemic medication.

Topical administration

Topical administration is the most common route and is appropriate for conditions affecting the adnexa, anterior chamber, iris and ciliary body. Posterior targets require systemic or intravitreal administration.

Agents for topical administration include aqueous solutions, suspensions, emulsions, gels and ointments. Agents are introduced to the conjunctival sac and mix with the tear film to be exposed to all corneal and conjunctival tissues. The degree of ocular penetration will depend upon drug concentration, pharmacokinetics in the conjunctival areas, corneal permeability and rate of elimination from the conjunctival sac. Solutions tend to be used in small animals, while ointments are often preferred in horses unless a device for improving the ease of administration (such as a sub-palpebral lavage system) is in place. For details of equine nursing see Chapter 8.

A standard drop contains 50 µl. This is far more than the eye can accommodate (the maximum volume which can be retained by the conjunctival sac in dogs is about 20 µl). The excess spills over the lids and drains down the nasolacrimal duct. Tear turnover is 1 µl/min and is increased by frequent blinking and greater lacrimation, both of which are stimulated further by the administration of topical medication! The half-life for drops in the eye is 3–6 minutes; thus, a minimum of 6 minutes should be left between drops. It is important to make sure that owners are aware that they should leave at least 6 minutes between different topical medications—usually 10–15 minutes is recommended otherwise the efficacy will be reduced. Clearly, when we consider the volume of a standard drop and the volume the eye can retain, it is obvious that one drop is sufficient and more than one only will increase wash-out times and may lessen the effect of the drug. Owners must be made aware of this fact. By elevating the animal's nose and occluding the ventral nasolacrimal punctum by pressing at the medial canthus, the clearance time can be prolonged.

Suspensions and emulsions increase drug availability for poorly soluble molecules such as corticosteroids. They should be gently shaken prior to use. Gels enhance viscosity and thus increase contact time (e.g. artificial tear gels). Ointments provide slow release so less frequent administration is needed, but they cause smearing and can encrust the lids. Owners often find ointments more difficult to apply, and tend to use too much. However, there is a balance to be found between ease of application and required frequency of administering medication. Often it is sensible to chose an ointment formulation for evening administration while using drops during the day. If corneal rupture has occurred (e.g. from a rapidly progressive ulcer), then ointment formulations are contraindicated.

The primary route of entry for topical medication is through the cornea, and a combination of lipophilic and hydrophilic parts of the drug molecule (i.e. both fat- and water-soluble) will enhance transport across the various corneal layers. If there is damage to the cornea (e.g. with ulceration), then agents tend to penetrate the eye more readily. Also with inflamed and diseased eyes, the absorption and effect of the drug might be heightened. Absorption also occurs through the conjunctiva. Agents are eliminated through the iridocorneal angle or by diffusion through uveal tissue and into drainage veins (uveoscleral outflow).

Application of topical medication

As mentioned previously, the conjunctival sac can only hold 20 µl yet the volume of a standard drop is 50 µl. Thus, one drop is ample and more than one will increase tear film turnover and flush the drug away. The bottle should be gently shaken (especially if a suspension is used) but not to excess since the formation of bubbles in the drops should be avoided. To apply drops, the animal's head should be elevated slightly using one hand to steady under the chin. The hand holding the bottle can rest on the animal's forehead from behind and a single drop is applied to the cornea or conjunctiva. By keeping in contact with the patient and coming from behind with the medication it is less likely that the animal will wriggle (Fig. 2.1a). Placing a finger across the medial canthus to occlude the nasolacrimal punctae will increase retention of the drug. The animal is allowed to blink and the head is kept elevated for a minute or so.

Ointments are similarly applied, although there is no need to occlude the punctae. A strip of ointment is placed on the cornea or conjunctiva and the lids manually closed to allow spread (Fig. 2.1b and Fig. 4.8, p. 60). Excess application will result in crusting of the lids and should be avoided. Owners often apply too much ointment and this can cause irritation.

If more than one topical agent is used a minimum of 6 minutes should elapse (ideally 10–15 minutes) and drops must always be applied before ointments.

Animals frequently want to rub following the administration of topical agents and should be distracted for a few minutes (e.g. taken for a walk, fed, groomed etc.). Some topical drops taste un-

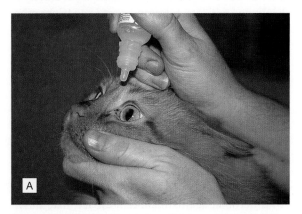
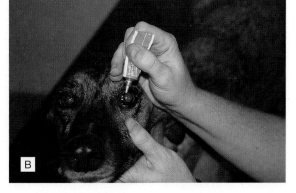

Fig. 2.1 Application of topical medication: a) drops; b) ointment.

pleasant when they drain down the nasolacrimal duct (e.g. atropine). This can cause hypersalivation and owners should be warned. The effect is lessened with the use of ointments.

If there are any special instructions regarding the storage of medications (e.g. refrigeration) the owners should be informed. Gloves should be worn when handling some medications, such as ciclosporin, steroids and chloramphenicol. Owners should also be made aware of how long they can use an opened bottle before discarding it; often this is a maximum of a month but can be less if no preservatives are included in the formulation (especially in single-use vials). It is important to ensure that owners have sufficient medication to last until their next visit, assuming that the patient will stay on medication until then. Often the containers are opaque and owners cannot tell when they are running low. The standard bottles are 5 ml and contain approximately 100 drops (assuming 20 drops per ml). So if both eyes are being medicated twice daily, a 5 ml bottle would be expected to last 25 days. However, owners can waste drops until they become proficient at medicating; thus we can assume that the bottle will last 3 weeks.

Local injections

Local injections bypass the need for diffusion across the cornea and provide a high concentration of active drug to the localised area. They are the method of choice for severe conditions. Four routes of administration are possible:

- subconjunctival
- intracameral (into the anterior chamber)
- intravitreal
- retrobulbar.

Subconjunctival injections are the most commonly used local injection. They are placed near the limbus in the bulbar conjunctiva following topical anaesthesia and sedation, or general anaesthesia. Subconjunctival injections are sometimes employed in fractious animals under sedation where topical medication cannot be applied, and are also used at the time of surgery to reduce the need for topical medication in the initial postoperative period. This is most common following cataract surgery. Other routes of local injection include intracameral (into the anterior chamber) and intravitreal. These routes are used by ophthalmic specialists under deep sedation or preferably general anaesthesia, and are the method of choice if treating severe intraocular infection or inflammation. Samples of aqueous or vitreous can be taken for laboratory investigation at the same time as the treatment is given. Retrobulbar injections can be used to deliver drugs directly to the orbital space, for example local anaesthetic agents. However, they carry significant risks of complication (including inadvertent globe penetration), and should only be used by ophthalmic specialists or anaesthetists.

Systemic medication

Systemic medication can be administered orally or by injection. It is effective for the treatment of eyelid diseases as well as those affecting the intraocular structures (such as uveitis or glaucoma) and retrobulbar conditions, including optic nerve disease. For many ocular problems a combination of both systemic and topical treatments is employed. The intraocular penetration of systemically administered drugs is dependent on their ability to cross the blood–ocular barrier. In a normal eye such agents need to be lipophilic. However, in most ocular diseases the blood–ocular barrier is compromised anyway such that many systemic agents can reach therapeutic levels in the eye regardless of their fat or water solubility. A disadvantage with systemic medication is that the entire body is exposed to the drug, and this can be significant, for example, in elderly or debilitated patients. It is important to consider other medications the patient is receiving since drug interactions could occur. Commonly used systemic agents include antibiotics, steroids, non-steroidal anti-inflammatory agents and anti-glaucoma agents.

PHARMACOLOGICAL AGENTS FOR OCULAR USE

Antimicrobial agents

Antimicrobial agents include antibacterial, antiviral and antifungal drugs.

Antibacterial agents

Both topical and systemic antibacterial agents are used in ocular conditions. Topical antibacterials are used for bacterial conjunctivitis, corneal inflammation (keratitis), corneal ulcers and uveitis. Systemic antibacterials are used for eyelid disease, posterior segment infections and retrobulbar problems.

The normal bacterial population of the ocular surface in both dogs and cats is a mixed selection of predominantly Gram-positive organisms. Thus, a broad-spectrum antibiotic agent is useful for primary bacterial conjunctivitis and corneal ulceration. Topical medication is usually applied 3–4 times daily, depending on the agent used, and for a period of 5–7 days. Details of various commonly used antibacterial agents are listed in Table 2.2.

Fortified antibacterial solutions are sometimes employed for serious or rapidly progressing ocular infections, such as melting corneal ulcers. They allow a rapid therapeutic drug concentration to be achieved and then maintained. Artificial tear solution is used as the base, and then antibiotics such as cephazolin or gentamicin can be added to achieve much higher concentrations than in commercially available solutions. These 'home-made' solutions are usually only stable for short periods (48 hours) and fresh solutions need to be made regularly.

Antiviral agents

Antiviral medications are used most commonly to treat feline herpes virus infections. They are most effective in the acute stage of disease. Several agents have been used such as trifluorothymidine, virabidine, idoxuridine and acyclovir. Trifluorothymidine seems to be the most beneficial in clinical cases, and it can be obtained as a topical preparation. Frequent administration is required initially (6–8 times daily for 3–5 days, then 4 times daily for 2–3 weeks until symptoms subside). Acyclovir (Zovirax, GSK) is used in humans for conditions caused by human herpes virus but seems to have little efficacy in the feline strain. Studies are ongoing to investigate the use of interferons for feline herpes virus. Certainly in humans they

can be helpful and have been shown to have a synergistic effect with acyclovir against feline herpes virus in cell cultures, although to date no clinical data are available to substantiate these findings.

L-Lysine is an amino acid. Oral L-Lysine has been advocated for feline herpes infections at a dose of 250–500 mg daily. It is thought to inhibit viral replication, although controlled studies have not yet been published regarding its efficacy in clinical cases. It can be obtained from health food shops.

Antifungal agents

Fungal infections are rare in the UK but are common in other parts of the world. In the UK they can occur in imported pets and seriously ill or immune-compromised patients. Topical and systemic antifungal agents are available. They should be chosen based on demonstration of the disease-causing organism (e.g. by cytology) and its likely sensitivity to the various agents. Ocular fungal infections can be limited to the eyelids, the cornea (usually with ulceration or stromal abscessation), or can be intraocular, either in isolation or following dissemination from a systemic fungal infection. Potential pathogens involved include *Aspergillus*, *Blastomyces*, *Coccidiodes* and *Cryptosporidium*. Drugs available for use include ketoconazole, natamycin, miconazole, clotrimazole and silver suphadiazine.

Anti-inflammatory drugs

Anti-inflammatory drugs are indicated for several ocular diseases where an immune-mediated component is present. These include chronic superficial keratitis, some types of keratoconjunctivitis sicca, allergic conjunctivitis and uveitis. For surface and anterior segment disease, topical corticosteroids and non-steroidal anti-inflammatory drugs (NSAIDs) are used, while their systemic counterparts are employed for severe intraocular inflammation. With cases of refractory or very severe intraocular inflammation, immunosuppressant agents are occasionally required. Although ocular inflammation is a protective mechanism, it

Table 2.2 Commonly used antibacterial agents (**topical** and systemic)

Drug type	Properties	Uses	Commercial products
b-lactam antibiotics—penicillins and cephalosporins	Bacteriocidal Excreted via kidneys Poor ocular penetration when given systemically unless BOB disrupted Topical agents will penetrate anterior chamber if cornea ulcerated Mostly Gram-positive activity	Aerobic infections of the orbit, eyelids and globe Cephalosporins safe for use in rabbits	Amoxicillin/clavulanic acid (Synulox, Pfizer) Cephalexin (Ceporex, Schering Plough; Cefaseptin, Vetoquinol among others) Cefazolin (Kefzol. Lilly)
Tetracyclines	Broad-spectrum Bacteriostatic Doxycyline has good ocular penetration unlike other tetracyclines Excreted via GI, biliary and urinary systems Good therapeutic levels in anterior chamber following topical administration	Chlamydophila *Mycoplasma* *Rickettsia*	Oxytetracycline—multiple systemic preparations Doxycycline (Ronaxan, Merial) **Chlortetracycline hydrochloride (Aureomycin ointment, Fort Dodge)**
Aminoglycocides	Bacteriocidal Excreted in urine Systemic agents do not cross BOB Gram-negative activity mainly Synergistic with penicillins	*Pseudomonas* spp. Melting corneal ulcers	**Gentamicin (Tiacil drops*, Virbac; Clinagel Vet, Janssen)** **Tobramycin (Tobrex, Alcon)** **Neomycin (often in combination with polymyxin and bacitracin e.g Neosporin drops, PLIVA)**
Macrolides and lincosamides	Usually Bacteriostatic Mainly Gram-positive activity Metabolised in the liver Good tissue penetration	*Toxoplasma gondii* Chlamydophila infections *Pseudomonas* *Pasteurella multocida*	Clindamycin (Antirobe, Pfizer) Azithromycin (Zithromax, Pfizer)
Fluoroquinolones	Bacteriocidal Broad-spectrum Some metabolism in liver before excretion via kidneys	*Pseudomonas* and other Gram-negative infections	Enfloxacillin, (Baytril, Bayer) (care in cats due to retinal degeneration at higher doses) Marbofloxacilin (Marbocyl, Vetoquinol) **Ciprofloxacin (Ciloxan, Alcon)** **Ofioxcicin (Exocin, Allergan)**

Table 2.2 Commonly used antibacterial agents (**topical** and systemic) *continued*

Drug type	Properties	Uses	Commercial products
Fusidic acid	Mainly Gram-positive with some Gram-negative activity Good corneal penetration	Gram-positive ocular surface disease, especially canine bacterial conjunctivitis	**Fusidic acid*** **(Fucithalmic, Leo)**
Chloramphenicol	Bacteriostatic Broad-spectrum Good corneal penetration and ocular penetration if used systemically	*Pasteurella multocida* Chlamydophila Prophylactically for ocular surgery	**Many products available, in systemic forms as well as drops and ointments**
Metronidazole	Bacteriocidal Good tissue penetration following systemic use	Anaerobic infections, e.g. retrobulbar or orbital disease	Several systemic preparations available
Polypeptide antibiotics	Bacteriocidal Do not penetrate cornea so restricted to surface disease Triple antibiotic provides broad-spectrum activity	Mixed ocular surface disease	**Combined preparations with polymyxin B, bacitracin and neomycin (Neosporin drops, PLIVA)**

Note: BOB = blood ocular barrier
*Licensed for use in rabbits
Topical medicines are in **bold**

can also cause significant intraocular damage, which in severe cases can lead to vision loss. It is for this reason it needs to be controlled with medication. However, it must be remembered that reducing the inflammatory response does not address the underlying cause which should also be treated whenever possible.

Corticosteroids

Corticosteroids for ocular use are glucocorticoids. They inhibit phospholipase which is a main enzyme in the inflammatory pathway and is responsible for the early step in the cascade leading to the production of the inflammatory mediators (mainly leukotrienes and prostaglandins) (Fig. 2.2). By blocking this pathway, glucocorticoids decrease vasodilation, capillary permeability, leukocyte proliferation and infiltration, and the cellular release of inflammatory mediators. They also inhibit the production of collagen by fibroblasts. However, they can have undesirable effects as well, including a reduction in corneal regeneration and the potentiation of corneal collagenase activity.

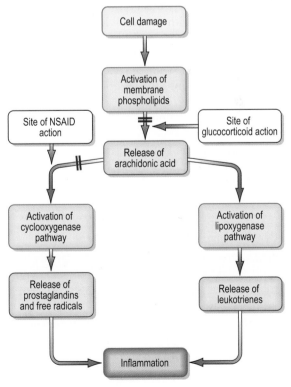

Fig. 2.2 The action of inflammatory mediators and the sites of action of anti-inflammatory agents.

For this reason, topical application is contra-indicated in the presence of corneal ulceration (corticosteroids can predispose to corneal melting and this can result in globe rupture necessitating enucleation). Long-term topical use in humans can result in both cataract formation and glaucoma; in cats, cataract formation has been reported following chronic systemic use but the risks are very small. Systemic changes which occur due to corticosteroid use include suppression of the pituitary–adrenal axis and hepatotoxity. Although mainly of concern with systemic use of these agents, some enzyme changes have been demonstrated following topical use and this must be considered in patients of low body weight.

Several topical glucocorticoid preparations are available for ocular use and are detailed in Table 2.3. They vary in their relative anti-inflammatory strengths and ability to penetrate the eye, and these two factors are considered when deciding which agent to use. Betamethasone and dexamethasone have the greatest potency, followed by fluoromethalone and prednisolone. The ability to cross the cornea depends on the lipid solubility of the base present with the steroid. Phosphate bases are water soluble (hydrophilic) so penetrate the cornea poorly and are used for surface disease, while preparations with an acetate base diffuse across the cornea into the anterior chamber easily and are the base of choice for anterior uveitis. In clinical practice, combined products with a corticosteroid and antibiotic are commonly used. They are of value when both bacterial infection and inflammation are present, and avoid the necessity

for multiple medications, but their use is probably over employed.

Subconjunctival corticosteroids are indicated for progressive, poorly responsive ocular inflammation, or if frequent topical administration cannot be achieved (due to lack of patient cooperation or owner compliance). Both short-acting agents, such as dexamethasone, and longer-acting products, like methyl prednisolone (Depo-Medrol Pharmacia and Upjohn), can be injected into the bulbar conjunctiva close to the limbus. They are useful to treat keratitis, episcleritis and anterior uveitis, and achieve therapeutic levels via diffusion through the conjunctiva and cornea as well as via the ciliary circulation. They are contraindicated in the presence of corneal ulceration in the same way as topical corticosteroids.

Systemic corticosteroids are recommended for severe anterior uveitis and posterior segment inflammation. If the blood ocular barriers have been compromised they readily penetrate the eye. Prednisolone and dexamethasone are the most commonly used agents.

Non-steroidal anti-inflammatory drugs (NSAIDs)

NSAIDs reduce the production of prostaglandins mainly by inhibiting the cyclo-oxygenase pathway of the inflammatory cascade (Fig. 2.2) They help to stabilise the blood–aqueous barrier, reduce miosis, decrease vasodilation and decrease vascular permeability. Although topical NSAIDS can be used in the face of corneal ulceration, unlike

Table 2.3 Topical corticosteroid (glucocorticoid) preparations

Generic name	Trade name	Indications
Betamethasone sodium phosphate 0.1%	Betnesol (Medeva)	Superficial ocular inflammation
Dexamethasone acetate 0.1% (in hypromellose)	Maxidex (Alcon)	Anterior uveitis
Fluoromethalone acetate 1.4% (in polyvinyl alcohol)	FML (Allergan)	Anterior uveitis and superficial ocular inflammation
Prednisolone acetate 1%	Predforte (Allergan)	Anterior uveitis
Prednisolone sodium phosphate 0.5%	Predsol (Medeva)	Superficial ocular inflammation

Table 2.4 Topical NSAIDs

Generic name	Trade name	Indications
Diclofenac sodium 0.1%	Voltarol Ophtha (CIBA Vision)	Cataract surgery
Flurbiprofen sodium 0.03%	Ocufen (Allergan)	Cataract surgery
Keratolac trometamol 0.5%	Acular (Allergan)	Anterior uveitis

corticosteroids, they do delay corneal epithelial healing to some extent so should be avoided if possible. Certainly their use in the face of ulceration should be carefully monitored by a specialist ophthalmologist. Topical agents should not be used in glaucoma since they can raise intraocular pressure and should also be used with caution if ocular haemorrhage is present (they decrease platelet aggregation and can promote intraocular haemorrhage). They are useful for postoperative pain relief and in the treatment of uveitis, both topically and systemically. Topical NSAIDs can be combined with topical corticosteroids where the effect of combining the agents may be additive. Topical NSAIDs are listed in Table 2.4. Systemic used drugs are commonly used as well and include carprofen (Rimadyl, Schering Plough) and meloxicam (Metacam, Boehringer Ingelheim).

Anti-allergy agents

Anti-allergy agents include topical mast cell stabilisers and antihistamines. They are used extensively for allergic conjunctivitis in humans and can be of some benefit in canine allergic conjunctivitis. None of these agents is licensed for veterinary use in the UK and their use should be limited to ophthalmic specialists.

Immunosuppressive agents

Ciclosporin is a potent immunosuppressive drug with a complicated mode of action. It is used topically (Optimmune, Schering Plough) for a variety of immune-mediated conditions such as keratoconjunctivitis sicca, chronic superficial keratitis, eosinophilic (proliferative) keratoconjunctivitis in cats and episcleritis. In addition to its immuno-suppressive effects, the drug stimulates tear production. Topically applied ciclosporin does not cross the cornea and is of no use in cases of anterior uveitis. It can be used systemically for severe inflammatory conditions, such as uveodermatological syndrome, but is very expensive. Systemic ciclosporin (Atopcia, Novartis) has recently become available in the UK but is currently only licensed for use in atopic dermatitis, so owners should be aware that its use for ophthalmic conditions is off-label.

Azathiaprine (Imuran, GlaxoWellcome) is a powerful immunosuppressive and cytotoxic agent and can be used systemically to treat severe autoimmune conditions, such as uveodermatological syndrome, severe panuveitis and episcleritis. It can be combined with systemic steroids. Potential side-effects include vomiting, diarrhoea, liver damage and severe bone marrow suppression. Regular haematology checks should be undertaken during the course of treatment (which is often long-term over months).

Anti-glaucoma drugs

Anti-glaucoma drugs, or ocular hypotensive agents, decrease the intraocular pressure by either reducing the rate of production of aqueous humour, or increasing its rate of outflow, or by both mechanisms. Many agents are available, which generally have been developed for human glaucoma, and their efficacy in canine and feline glaucoma can be disappointing. Side-effects in dogs and cats especially can be significant with some human preparations. Multiple classes of drug are available, but those which are most useful for our patients include carbonic anhydrase inhibitors, osmotic diuretics and prostaglandin analogues. Parasympathomimetics and adrenergic agents are

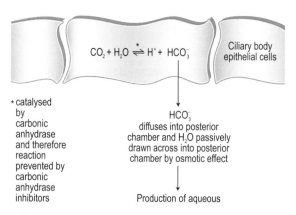

$$CO_2 + H_2O \overset{*}{\rightleftharpoons} H^+ + HCO_3^-$$

Ciliary body epithelial cells

* catalysed by carbonic anhydrase and therefore reaction prevented by carbonic anhydrase inhibitors

HCO_3^- diffuses into posterior chamber and H_2O passively drawn across into posterior chamber by osmotic effect

Production of aqueous

Fig. 2.3 Aqueous production and activity of carbonic anhydrase inhibitors in the ciliary body epithelium.

less useful, despite being frequently prescribed for people with glaucoma.

Carbonic anhydrase inhibitors reduce the production of aqueous humour. Their site of action is the ciliary body, where they prevent the formation of bicarbonate ions from water and carbon dioxide in the epithelium of the ciliary processes (Fig. 2.3). The bicarbonate ions combine with sodium and pass into the posterior chamber, bringing water with them. By reducing the production of bicarbonate ions, the inhibition of the enzyme carbonic anhydrase leads to less water passing into the posterior chamber and, therefore, a lowering of intraocular pressure. Systemic carbonic anhydrase inhibitors, such as acetazolamide (Diamox, Wyeth), have common side-effects, including nausea, anorexia, depression, vomiting and diarrhoea and increased rates of respiration. Their use in cats is particularly limited due to these adverse effects. Systemic carbonic anhydrase inhibitors have been largely superseded by the topical agents, such as dorzolamide (Trusopt, MSD) and brinzolamide (Azopt, Allergan). They can be used long-term to control glaucoma, often in combination with other agents. They can be used in both dogs and cats but seem to be more efficacious in the former.

Osmotic diuretics are used in the emergency treatment for acute glaucoma, and intravenous mannitol is the drug of choice. Oral glycerol (glycerine) can also be given and has the advantage that owners can keep this at home for emergency use. The administration of either osmotic diuretic leads to a rapid reduction in intraocular pressure as water is removed from the aqueous and vitreous. Unfortunately, their effects are only short-acting (up to 5 hours). Once they have reduced the intraocular pressure, more long-term measures to control the glaucoma, such as surgery or a medical management regime, can be arranged. They should not be used in patients with renal insufficiency as they can trigger renal failure following the hypovolaemia they induce. Thus routine blood biochemistry and urine samples should be taken prior to their administration. Mannitol is usually given at a dose rate of 5–10 ml/kg of a 20% solution over a 20–30 minute period, and intraocular pressure is measured on an hourly, or more frequent, basis.

Prostaglandin analogues lower intraocular pressure by increasing the outflow of aqueous from the anterior chamber. Ocular penetration is achieved by the lipophilic ester attached to the prostaglandin molecule itself, since the latter is unable to cross the cornea. Latanoprost 0.005% (Xalatan, Pharmacia and Upjohn) or bimatoprost 0.03% (Lumigan, Allergan) can be used once or twice daily in canine glaucoma cases, often in combination with a topical carbonic anhydrase inhibitor. These agents are contraindicated if uveitis is present. A profound miosis can be induced which can result in tunnel vision in some patients.

Other anti-glaucoma drugs include parasympathomimetics, such as pilocarpine which increases aqueous outflow (so long as the drainage angle is still functional), and beta-blockers such as timolol maleate which reduces aqueous production. Although very useful in human glaucoma, these agents are of little use in canine and feline glaucoma.

Mydriatic and cycloplegic agents

Mydriatic agents dilate the pupil and are used for diagnostic as well as therapeutic purposes. The pupil needs to be dilated to perform a full ophthalmic examination of the lens and fundus, and to be able to carry out certain intraocular operations such as cataract surgery. If uveitis is present, a dilated pupil is beneficial since it reduces the incidence of adhesion formation (synechiae) between the iris and lens (posterior) or the iris and cornea (anterior synechiae). Cycloplegic agents relax the ciliary body musculature, which also results in pupil dilation, and are used in cases of anterior uveitis to relieve the ciliary spasm, which causes a painful miosis (pupil constriction). Mydriatics, such as phenylephrine and adrenaline, are sympathomimetic in action and act directly to stimulate the dilator muscle of the pupil, while parasympatholytics, such as atropine and tropicamide, block the iris sphincter and ciliary body muscles. As such, parasympatholytic agents are both mydriatic and cycloplegic, while sympathomimetics only produce pupil dilation.

The most frequently used agents are tropicamide (0.1% and 1% Mydriacyl, Alcon) and atropine sulphate 1% (various products available in both drop and ointment formulations). Tropicamide is used mainly for diagnostic purposes, has a rapid onset (20 minutes) and lasts for several hours. Atropine has a slower onset but longer duration of action, especially in a non-inflamed eye. It is applied several times daily to achieve mydriasis and then as frequently as required to maintain the pupil dilation (usually once or twice daily). It should be used with care if tear production is reduced (since it reduces tear production even further), and it must not be used in glaucoma cases in dogs and cats since it will further increase intraocular pressure. Atropine has a bitter taste and can cause salivation after topical application, as the drug drains down the nasolacrimal ducts into the mouth. Owners should be warned of this. Ointments cause less of a problem and are the formulation of choice in cats.

Sympathomimetics, such as phenylephrine, can be used in severe uveitis where the miosis is profound since they act synergistically with atropine and thus the likelihood of producing some pupil dilation is increased. They are also used to assist the localisation of lesions in Horner's syndrome, a neurological disorder where there is disruption of the sympathetic nerve supply to the eye.

Tear stimulants and substitutes

Tear stimulants increase tear production and are the treatment of choice for keratoconjunctivitis sicca (dry eye), especially if due to immune-mediated disease. Ciclosporin (0.2% ciclosporin, Optimmune, Schering Plough) is available as an ointment and is generally used twice daily. Improvements in Schirmer tear test readings can be expected in 2–6 weeks. Long-term medication, often for life, is required to control the dry eye. Pilocarpine can also be an effective tear stimulant, providing some functional lacrimal tissue is present. It can be used topically or, more commonly, orally in the food twice daily and is of particular value in cases of neurogenic keratoconjunctivitis sicca. Dose rates are empirical and depend on the response (and presence of side-effects) in each individual. However, 1 drop/5 kg of 2% pilocarpine, twice daily, is often used initially.

Tear substitutes (lacrimomimetics) are used in the treatment of keratoconjunctivitis sicca, often in combination with ciclosporin. These artificial tears moisten and lubricate the dry ocular surfaces, and many different types exist. Aqueous formulations, gels and ointments are available. Aqueous formulations require very frequent application and for this reason their use is limited in our patients. Gel formulations containing carbomer 980 (Viscotears, CIBA vision, GelTears, Chauvin) are longer lasting and require 4–6 times daily application. They also have mucin-like properties which help to provide a smooth optical surface as well as lubricating the tissues. Ointment formulations such as liquid paraffin (Lacrilube, Allergan) have good ocular retention and mimic the lipid layer of the precorneal tear film. They are often applied at night. They are also useful as ocular protectants during anaesthesia, or if blinking cannot occur due to facial nerve paralysis or other causes. More recently introduced tear replacement agents include viscoelastic solutions, such as hyaluronic acid and chondroitin sulphate, and these are being used in canine keratoconjunctivitis sicca with variable success.

Topical anaesthetic agents

Topical anaesthetics interrupt the sensory innervation to the cornea or conjunctiva. Local injections of anaesthetic agents can also be used to block the sensory or motor innervation and are used more in large animals than in dogs and cats. Examples of local anaesthesia include auriculo-palpebral, supraorbital and retrobulbar blocks. Topical anaesthetics are used to assist the examination of a painful eye, for diagnostic tests such as tonometry, gonioscopy and ocular ultrasonography, and for taking conjunctival biopsy samples. They can also be used when examining animals with entropion (in-turning eyelids) to assess the anatomic versus spastic component of the condition. This is discussed further in Chapter 7. Proxymetacaine (proparacaine) and amethocaine (tetracaine) are the most commonly used products. They are effective in 2–3 minutes and last for about 20 minutes. They must not be used to treat painful eyes as they damage the corneal epithelium and slow healing. They should not be instilled prior to sample collection for bacterial culture since they can have an antimicrobial effect. For conjunctival anaesthesia it is useful to soak a cotton bud with the topical anaesthetic and then hold this against the area to be desensitised for a minute or so. Sufficient anaesthesia is produced to allow biopsy samples or to trim conjunctival pedicle grafts using this technique.

Ophthalmic dyes

Fluorescein is the most commonly used ophthalmic dye. It is an orange colour in solution and on the frequently encountered impregnated paper strips (Fluorets strips (Chauvin)), but changes to bright green in alkaline conditions such as saline solutions or the tear film. It does not stain the intact corneal epithelium since it is not lipid-soluble, but if any ulceration is present it will rapidly adhere to the exposed hydrophilic stroma. The area of ulceration will be delineated and tiny areas will be detected more efficiently using blue light if magnification is not available. It is important to flush away excess dye to prevent false positive readings (e.g. if the corneal surface is irregular). Fluorescein can also be used to assess the patency of the nasolacrimal system, as dye should appear at the ipsilateral nostril or in the mouth following topical ocular application.

Rose Bengal is a deep pink dye which stains dead and devitalised epithelium. Like fluorescein it is available in both solution and impregnated paper strips. It is mainly used to detect the fine branching ulcers (dendritic) seen in acute feline herpes virus infections. These ulcers are very shallow and do not always stain positive with fluorescein. The application of rose Bengal causes slight irritation so it should be thoroughly flushed from the eye with sterile saline solution. Historically, it has also been used in the diagnosis of keratoconjunctivitis sicca but is rarely used for this nowadays.

Specialist ophthalmic agents

In this section we will briefly consider some products used in specialised ophthalmic practice. These include anticollagenase agents, fibrinolytic products, antifibrotic agents, viscoelastic materials, tissue glue, intraocular irrigating solutions and ocular disinfectants.

Anticollagenase agents

Anticollagenase agents can be helpful for treating melting ulcers. A melting ulcer is a true ocular emergency and aggressive treatment is necessary to salvage the eye. Excessive collagenase activity occurs which causes the breakdown of the corneal stroma and a rapidly deepening ulcer. The collagenase activity comes from a combination of exogenous bacterial and endogenous sources—neutrophils and dying corneal stromal cells. Drugs which reduce collagenase activity can help to stabilise the cornea. Sodium or potassium EDTA, acetylcysteine and autologous serum (from a centrifuged blood sample) can all be employed. The efficacy of these compounds is questionable but they certainly seem to assist with the arrest of corneal degradation in some cases. Autologous serum is the easiest to obtain but must be kept in conditions of strict asepsis since it is an ideal bacterial culture medium. It is generally administered every 1–2 hours to hospitalised patients, and a fresh sample should be collected on a daily basis.

Fibrinolytic agents

Fibrinolytic agents, such as tissue-type plasminogen activator (tPA), are useful in specialist oph-

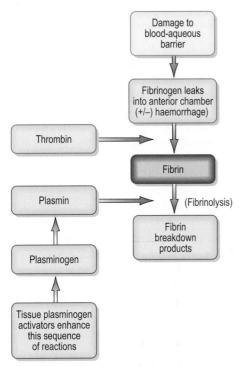

Fig. 2.4 The formation and breakdown of fibrin.

thalmic practice. They dissolve blood and fibrin clots in the anterior chamber if injected directly into the anterior chamber (under general anaesthesia). This is of use since the presence of clots will reduce visual clarity and contribute to synechia formation (adhesions) together with increasing the risk of secondary glaucoma development. Haemorrhage or leakage of serum proteins from a damaged blood–aqueous barrier leads to the formation of fibrinogen in the anterior chamber. This is converted to fibrin by the action of thrombin. Fibrin is broken down by plasmin, which in turn is activated by plasminogen. Thus, a plasminogen activator enhances fibrinolysis (Fig. 2.4). The most widely used agent is human recombinant tPa, although other products available include streptokinase and urokinase. The standard dose is 25 µg tPa. This is diluted from the standard human dose vials (of 20 mg, 50 mg or 100 mg) and stored in 100 µL aliquots in a $-70\,^{\circ}$C freezer until needed. Once injected, the clots start to dissolve within 15–30 minutes.

Antifibrotic agents

Antifibrotic agents, such as mitomycin C and 5-fluorouracil, inhibit fibroplasia and are used following glaucoma implant surgery. They reduce the amount of scar tissue and aim to maintain implant function for longer. They are routinely employed in human surgery, but their efficacy in canine cases is still being investigated. Since these agents reduce fibroblast proliferation and are extremely potent, extreme caution must be taken if using them. Inadvertently applying them in the wrong place could result in severe corneal ulceration and wound breakdown.

Viscoelastic agents

Viscoelastic agents are used during intraocular surgery. They separate the tissues, help maintain a formed globe and protect delicate tissues from instrument tips and vibrations from the phaco-emulsification handpiece, and cushion against turbulence from irrigating fluids during surgery. They are essential for phacoemulsification and intraocular lens implantation and are useful for maintaining the anterior chamber during the removal of perforating or intraocular foreign bodies. Many products are available and surgeon preference will decide the agent to be used. They vary according to viscosity (i.e. the ability to flow). High-viscosity agents will maintain a formed anterior chamber better than low-viscosity agents but will be more difficult to inject and remove. Other parameters which contribute to the behaviour of the agent include elasticity, plasticity, cohesiveness and coatability. Commonly used products include sodium hyaluronate, which is very viscous, elastic and cohesive, and chondroitin sulphate, which has better coating ability but is less viscous. The two agents can be combined in commercially available products. Hydroxypropyl methylcellulose is a much cheaper alternative but is much less viscous.

Tissue adhesives

Tissue adhesives are recommended for the treatment of some corneal ulcers and lacerations.

N-butyl cyanoacrylate is most widely used. Corneal surfaces must be thoroughly dry before the glue is applied and the patient must be adequately restrained either by sedation and topical anaesthesia or general anaesthesia. A tiny aliquot of glue is placed onto the ulcer using a 25 gauge needle on a 0.5 mL or tuberculin syringe. It takes up to a minute for the glue to polymerise and no blinking should occur during this time. The placement of a bandage contact lens will promote patient comfort since the surface of the glue can be quite rough. The glue will slough off as the ulcer heals or can be removed with a pair of fine forceps.

Intraocular irrigating solutions and ocular disinfectants

Intraocular irrigating solutions are usually balanced salt solutions. The addition of bicarbonate and glutathione provides better protection to the corneal endothelium and is advised during phacoemulsification (BSS Plus, Alcon). Irrigating solutions must be isotonic, non-irritating and have a physiological pH. During cataract surgery some surgeons include adrenaline and heparin in their irrigating fluids to assist pupil dilation and as an anti-coagulant, respectively.

Ocular disinfectants are used prior to any surgery to the adnexa, cornea or intraocular structures. Surgical preparation of the eye is discussed further in Chapter 5. Povidine iodine is considered the disinfectant of choice. It kills most bacteria within a minute, but takes slightly longer for fungal spores. Solutions must be used and not scrub preparations since these will damage the corneal and conjunctival tissues. Dilutions of 1:10 to 1:50 are recommended. Re-colonisation by bacteria is inhibited for 60 minutes following a careful surgical preparation with dilute povidine iodine solution.

PHARMACY MANAGEMENT

A detailed review of the legislation regarding the storage, prescription and dispensing of drugs is beyond the scope of this text. However, there are certain points which should be mentioned. It is essential that medicines are stored according to the manufacturer's recommendations. For some ocular preparations this involves refrigeration and even freezing (e.g. aliquots of tissue plaminogen activator, tPa). As such, fridge thermometers should be routinely checked and both maximum and minimum thermometers should be used. Proper stock control is mandatory, with the oldest stock being used first, and use-by dates should always be checked prior to dispensing medications. Some ocular products are available without prescription and owners can obtain these wherever they like (e.g. tear substitutes and saline solutions). Prescription-only medications can be veterinary but many are human products. In the UK, a veterinary medicine may only be administered to an animal if it has a product licence for the treatment of that particular condition in that particular species. However, since for many ocular diseases there is no licensed product available for any animal species for the condition in question (e.g. glaucoma), it is acceptable to use a licensed human product.

All products dispensed to owners must be correctly packaged and labelled. It is important to go through the dosing instructions with owners and to ensure that they are competent at medicating their pet. Owners should also be made aware if items should be kept in the fridge, and how long a product can be used once opened. This is usually a month for topical products. Owners should be encouraged to return any unused medications to the surgery for correct disposal.

BIBLIOGRAPHY AND FURTHER READING

Bishop Y, ed. The veterinary formulary 6th edn. London: Pharmaceutical Press; 2004.

Gelatt KN. Veterinary ophthalmology. 3rd edn. Philadelphia: Lippincott Williams & Wilkins; 1999.

Lane DR, Cooper B, eds. Veterinary nursing. 3rd edn. Oxford: Butterworth Heinemann; 2003.

Petersen-Jones S, Crispin S, eds. BSAVA manual of small animal ophthalmology. 2nd edn. Gloucester: British Small Animal Veterinary Association; 2002.

3 Ophthalmic examination including diagnostic tests

CHAPTER SUMMARY

- Introduction
- History taking
- The ophthalmic examination
- Further diagnostic tests
  - Ophthalmic dyes
  - Nasolacrimal duct investigation
  - Tonometry
  - Gonioscopy
  - Electroretinography
  - Blood pressure measurement
- Laboratory investigation
- Ocular imaging

INTRODUCTION

A routine ophthalmic examination should be performed on all animals presenting with an ocular complaint. An experienced nurse can be of great help to the veterinary ophthalmologist—history taking, certain diagnostic tests, such as vision assessment and Schirmer tear test readings, and sampling, such as taking swabs for culture and sensitivity, can all be performed by nurses. It is important for you to understand the principles of the ophthalmic examination in order to assist the clinician and anticipate their requirements such

that the examination is conducted smoothly and is as stress-free as possible for the patient.

To perform an ophthalmological examination it is mandatory to have a quiet examination room which can be fully darkened. For this discussion we will concentrate only on small animal patients. However, the same principles apply to horses and farm species. Any differences or special precautions required for the examination of horses are discussed in the section on equine nursing in Chapter 8. It is useful if the examination table can be varied in height. Large dogs can be examined on the floor but it is often easier to examine medium-sized dogs (e.g. Labrador retriever) and smaller breeds on a table. Cats should be allowed a few minutes to acclimatise themselves in the room before being handled. The facilities and instruments required for an ocular examination are listed in Table 3.1. Disposables needed for the ophthalmic examination are listed in Table 3.2.

HISTORY TAKING

History taking can be divided into general history and that specifically pertaining to the eyes. A general history should consider the following points:

- **Breed.** Pedigree dogs and cats can suffer from inherited eye diseases and so identifying the breed is of significant importance. Even in

Table 3.1 Facilities and equipment required for ophthalmic examination

General practice	Ophthalmology practice
• Room capable of being fully darkened	• All equipment as listed for general practice
• Table of adjustable height	• Slit lamp biomicroscope
• Pen torch	• Finhoff transilluminator
• Direct ophthalmoscope	• Indirect ophthalmoscope
• Magnifying lens	• Goniolens
• Magnifying loupes	
• Tonometer	

Table 3.2 Disposables required for ophthalmic examination

- Schirmer tear test papers
- Fluorescein paper test strips
- Rose Bengal dye *
- Cotton wool and gauze swabs
- Tropicamide 1% (Mydriacyl, Alcon)
- Topical anaesthetic (Proxymetacaine)
- Sterile saline
- Lacrimal cannulae
- Bacterial swabs and transport media
- Slides and laboratory equipment

*For specialty ophthalmology practice

crossbred dogs, the general type of dog might be relevant. For example, terriers are prone to lens luxation, which is seen in pedigree wire haired fox terriers and miniature bull terriers among others, but is also common in all types of Jack Russell from the pedigree Parson terrier to the general terrier-type. In cats, corneal sequestrum is a common condition in Persians and Burmese, while retinal degeneration is recognised in Siamese and Abyssinian breeds. Obviously, we must not jump to conclusions and assume that just because we have a boxer dog with a sore eye it must have a non-healing corneal ulcer, but common things are commonest and breed predispositions are particularly important in ophthalmology.

- **Age.** This is always a factor to be considered. Conditions such as entropion and prolapse of the nictitans gland (cherry eye) are common in young animals (3–12 months), while neoplasia is more common in older patients. Congenital problems such as cataract can be detected in young animals, although sometimes these are not noticed until later in life.

- **Sex.** Although of less importance with regard to ophthalmology than for some other specialties, the sex of the patient might have some influence on its ocular disease. For example, young male dogs are more prone to entropion, and keratoconjunctivitis sicca is seen in neutered females more commonly than entire males.

- **General health.** Many ocular conditions can be manifestations of systemic disease, and questions related to appetite, general demeanour and concurrent illness are extremely important. Examples might include the dog with diabetes mellitus which presents with sudden-onset blindness due to cataract formation, or a cat with retinal haemorrhages which has systemic hypertension.

- **Medications administered.** Previous or ongoing medication may be the cause of some ophthalmic conditions. An example is the dog with colitis which is treated with salazopyrin and develops an acute, severe bilateral keratoconjunctivitis sicca. Some ophthalmic drugs can cause a localised hypersensitivity which exacerbates the ocular disease. Owners are notorious for using left-over medication from a previous problem—for example, treating a sore eye with a steroid drop that their mother used last year after her cataract operation, only to discover that the dog has a sore eye due to a corneal ulcer and the 'self-medication' has only made things worse. This situation is unfortunately commonly encountered.

- **Presence of other pets in the house.** This is particularly relevant when considering infectious diseases such as feline herpes virus where repeated infection can be a problem. If the owner has more than one pet, it is important to find out if others are affected. The presence of a new puppy in a home with a cat might be relevant if the puppy is brought to the surgery with an acutely painful eye—it is quite likely that the cat has scratched it!

- **Source of the pet.** Cats from rescue centres and/or breeders may have pre-existing diseases such as herpes or *Chlamydophila* infections, while dogs from puppy farms may be prone to inherited ocular disease since control measures to prevent these are rarely followed.
- **Travel history.** This is becoming more and more relevant in the UK since the introduction of the Pets Passports schemes, but is also relevant in all countries. Several Mediterranean diseases, such as Leishmania and Erlichia, have ocular involvement, while some fungal conditions are found in certain US states but not others.

Once we have taken a thorough general history we can move on to the more specific ophthalmic history. This will include asking the owners the following questions:

- What was the first thing the owner noticed wrong with the eye(s)? Were they concerned about discharge, pain, redness or other change in colour, an alteration in appearance of the eye (e.g. bulging or sunken), or perhaps they noted a decrease in vision?
- When did they notice something wrong? The time span of the disease is very relevant. Some owners will bring a pet along to the surgery immediately, while it is always surprising how some will do nothing for a considerable period of time!
- Progression of the problem: has the problem become worse, better or stayed the same since it was first noticed? Has it been present continuously or intermittently and, if the latter, has the owner noticed any 'trigger factor' which brought on a return of the symptoms? For example, did the atopic Labrador retriever always have itchy eyes when he returned from a walk through certain fields, which could suggest an allergic component.
- Is the problem unilateral or bilateral? As mentioned in the general history taking, systemic disease may be the underlying problem and this is much more likely with bilateral conditions. With infectious disease we might also expect a bilateral presentation, although it is not unusual for one eye to be affected before the other. *Chlamydophila* in cats is an example

where a delay of a few days can be seen before the second eye develops symptoms.

- Treatment: has the owner given any medication. If so, what was the medication, and was it beneficial or detrimental?
- Previous ocular history: it is important to establish whether the pet has had any ocular problem in the past and, if so, was the presentation the same and was the same eye previously affected. Also, response to treatment given previously is relevant.

Hands-off examination

Once a careful history has been taken, the first part of any ophthalmic examination begins with observation of the patient. This can actually be done while taking the history from the owner. Dogs are allowed to wander off the lead and investigate the consulting room while cats are encouraged out of their baskets and then watched from a distance. It is important to look at the behaviour of the pet, along with the gross appearance of the eyes and face. Look for:

- Signs of ocular discomfort—blepharospasm (squinting), increased lacrimation or other discharge.
- Symmetry of the eyes and face—sunken or small eyes, enlargement of the globe, periorbital swellings or squints.
- Clues that the animal has been rubbing—periorbital hair loss and erythema (redness) could suggest this, as could saliva staining on the front legs where the animal licks then rubs the face.

Basic assessment of the visual ability of the patient can be undertaken at this time. Blind animals will often stay close to the owner and not move around the room, while if they do move they are often very cautious, sniffing the environment and exhibiting a high-stepping gait.

How to hold the patient for examination

The patient can now be gently restrained for the next stage of the ophthalmological examination. Lightly holding under the chin helps to keep the

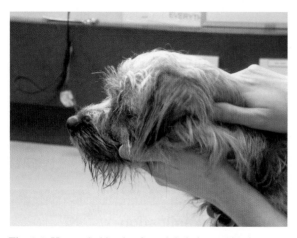

Fig. 3.1 How to hold a dog for ophthalmic examination.

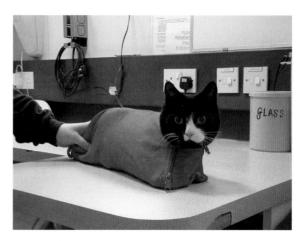

Fig. 3.3 Cat bag for restraint of fractious cats.

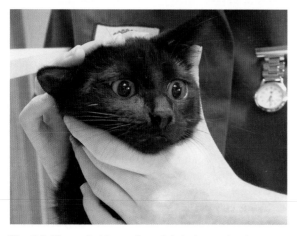

Fig. 3.2 How to hold a cat for ophthalmic examination.

head straight. The second hand can gently rest behind the animal's head to prevent it from drawing back from the examination lights. In general, minimal restraint is best—the animal is less likely to struggle and get stressed. Holding the front legs above the elbow to prevent the patient from pawing or scratching the ophthalmologist is useful and can be done when the ophthalmologist is holding the patient's head themselves. Calm reassurance of the patient is advised. With this approach, most dogs and cats can be easily examined. Figures 3.1 and 3.2 are examples of how to hold dogs and cats.

Confidence by both the nurse and the veterinary surgeon will go a long way towards relaxing the patient. However, some patients need to be muzzled and sometimes it is necessary to resort to wrapping cats in towels or cat-bags to examine them (Fig. 3.3). Care must be taken to avoid 'scruffing' the patient. This will alter the position of the eyelids and periocular skin, and can predispose to traumatic proptosis in brachycephalic breeds. Sedation or general anaesthesia is sometimes required, but ophthalmic examination of such patients is difficult and often unrewarding.

Hands-on examination

The first part of the hands-on examination takes place in a well-lit room. It is useful to have an ophthalmic examination form to fill out during the examination (Fig. 3.4). This will form an accurate record of the examination and ensure that no part of the examination is overlooked. Photographs can also be taken for records.

A close inspection of the gross appearance of the eyes and face is performed with illumination using a pen torch to highlight particular structures. Particular things to consider include the presence of any ocular discharge—the nature and amount, and whether unilateral or bilateral. Some dogs commonly have a small amount of mucoid discharge at the medial canthus, especially those with doliocephalic conformation, such as Dobermans. This can be considered a normal finding in these breeds, whereas a copious green-yellow, pus-like discharge is certainly not! The size of both eyes should be compared. They should be symmetrical, but if not it is necessary to establish whether one is enlarged (hydrophthalmic) or the

OPHTHALMOLOGY EXAMINATION

Owners name.. Animal name..................................
Address... Breed..
.... Age..................... Sex..............
......................................Postcode.......................
DATE...

Referring Vet..
....
....
.... INS.......................
Phone..........................Fax....................................

History & Clinical exam...…
....……
....……
....……
....……

RIGHT	**LEFT**
Menace yes / no	**Menace** yes / no
PLR Direct ☐ Consensual ☐	☐ Direct **PLR** ☐ Consensual
STT .... mm/min	STT .... mm/min
IOP .... mm/Hg	IOP .... mm/Hg
Gonioscopy	Gonioscopy

Mydriatic ☐   ☐   time ....

O   info sheet given

Diagnosis..Prognosis....................................
Treatment...
....
....
Re-examination...

Fig. 3.4 Sample eye examination form.

other is shrunken (microphthalmic). In addition to size, the actual position of the eyes should be noted. Looking from above the patient directly down on the head can assist in establishing the presence of exophthalmos (protruded eye), enophthalmos (sunken eye) or strabismus (squint). It is essential to differentiate between hydrophthalmos and exophthalmos, for example. General head symmetry and the presence of periorbital swellings should also be considered.

It might be necessary to take samples for laboratory analysis at this stage if indicated. Swabs for bacterial culture and isolation should be taken before any discharges are cleaned away. These procedures will be discussed in greater detail later in this chapter.

Schirmer tear test readings

Schirmer tear test readings should be taken before the eyes are cleaned or handled further. Commercial tear testing strips are used (colour bar calibrated strips are the easiest to use and are available from Schering Plough). The strips come in sterile plastic wallets. The strips should be bent at the notch while still in their plastic wallet (to prevent sweat and grease from hands interfering with the readings). The packet is opened and each test paper is held at the distal end (away from the notch). The shorter piece is placed in the ventral conjunctival sac $^{1}/_{2}$ to $^{2}/_{3}$ along from the medial canthus (i.e. out of the way of the third eyelid; see Fig. 3.5). The strip is left in position for one minute before removing and immediately reading the level of wetting on the scale. It is easier to hold the patient's eye closed to prevent the strip from falling out prematurely. Topical anaesthetics are not used prior to measurement. The readings

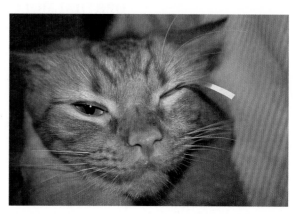

Fig. 3.5 Schirmer tear test being performed in a cat.

obtained can be interpreted following the guidelines listed in Table 3.3.

Basic vision testing and neurological tests

1. Menace response

A threatening gesture will cause the animal to blink and pull away slightly (Fig. 3.6). This reflex tests the visual pathway (optic nerve, cranial nerve II) and the ability to close the lids (facial nerve, cranial nerve VII), i.e. can the animal see you and if so can it react and blink normally. It is important that the stimulus is visual only, and does not generate air currents which would trigger sensory nerve endings on the cornea and skin (trigeminal nerve, cranial nerve V). For this reason, some people advocate testing from behind a clear Perspex screen, but in reality this is not really necessary. So long as the hand movements involve just a couple of fingers rather than waving the whole hand in front

Table 3.3 Schirmer tear test readings in dogs and cats		
	Dog	**Cat**
Normal	15–25 mm/min	Readings variable and often lower than in the dog, especially in stressed cats
Borderline	10–15 mm/min	
Keratoconjunctivitis sicca (KCS)	< 10 mm/min	

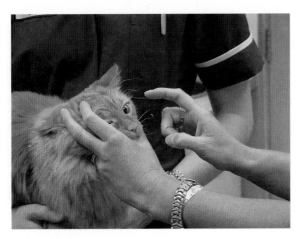

Fig. 3.6 Menace response.

of the eyes there should not be any confusion over the actual reflex being tested. It is important to stimulate both from directly in front of the eyes and also from other angles—above and below, medial and lateral. The fellow eye can be covered with your other hand to assess each eye separately.

A couple of points need considering in interpretation of the menace response. If the animal is visual but cannot blink (e.g. with facial nerve paralysis), the third eyelid will move across the globe and the animal will pull back from the stimulus. A palpebral reflex can then be performed to confirm that the animal cannot blink (see below). However, it is clear that it could see, and react to, the menacing gesture. Blind animals will not react at all. Another very important point to remember is that the menace response is a learned response and not present in very young animals (one reason why young puppies are often scratched on the cornea by the family cat; they have not learned to blink for protection).

2. Dazzle reflex

A very bright light source is needed for this test (e.g. a Finhoff transilluminator or slit lamp biomicroscope on maximum intensity). Often a pen torch is not bright enough. The animal is seen to blink and sometimes pull away when the bright light is shone into each eye in turn. This tests the same two nerves as the menace response (optic and facial nerves), but unlike the menace response it does not require involvement of the cerebral cortex for the reflex to occur. It is a useful test if the retina and optic nerve cannot be examined due to opacity in the eye (e.g. cataract). A positive reflex suggests that the retina and optic nerve are functional.

3. Tracking responses (cotton wool balls)

Cotton wool is used because it does not smell strongly and makes no sound when it lands. Thus, we can be sure that we are testing vision and not smell or hearing instead! Several small pieces are used and dropped from above the animal's face once you have gained their attention. Dogs and cats have better movement detection than us and should follow the path of the falling cotton wool. Each eye can be tested separately and the test can be performed in bright and dim lighting conditions (some diseases cause night blindness and in these circumstances the animals respond normally in the bright light but fail to react in the dim light). False negative results are seen when the animals are bored or disinterested (more of a problem in cats). Sometimes dangling a loose piece of bandage will encourage the cat to 'track' the movement.

4. Maze testing

An unfamiliar room is used (e.g. a large consulting room or empty waiting room). A mixture of solid objects (e.g. bins) and open objects (e.g. chairs) is chosen and randomly placed in the room (Fig. 3.7). The animal is held at one corner of the room while the owner stands at the other side of the room and then calls to the pet. Normally sighted animals will negotiate the room confidently, but visually impaired ones will be hesitant and slow, and may bump into objects. This test should be performed in both bright and dim lighting levels and the objects should be moved about in between tests. It can be difficult to get cats to co-operate. The test can be adapted for them by placing their basket on the floor behind a chair and watching to see how they manage to get to the safety of their basket!

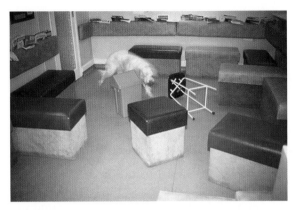

Fig. 3.7 Maze test—the confident visual dog rapidly moves around the obstacles.

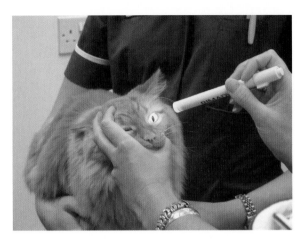

Fig. 3.8 Pupillary light reflex tested using a pen torch.

5. Palpebral (blink) reflex

It is important to check that the animal can blink normally. Sensory stimulation of the trigeminal nerve (cranial nerve V) by tapping the medial and lateral canthal skin should result in a brisk closing of the eyelids (facial nerve, cranial nerve VII). The animal may also try to move away. If the animal cannot feel the stimulation then it will not blink (but should have a normal menace response assuming that it can see). If the animal can feel the stimulus but cannot blink due to a facial nerve paralysis, it is likely to move away from the stimulus and would have an abnormal menace response where the third eyelid crosses the cornea but no blink occurs, as mentioned previously. Corneal sensitivity can also be tested by touching the corneal surface with a wisp of cotton wool and watching a normal blink. It is usually very difficult to touch the cornea in this way without the animal trying to blink.

6. Pupillary light reflexes

Pupillary light reflexes should be assessed both in normal room light and in the dark. They are more sensitive in the dark. It should be remembered that these are not an assessment of vision but an indication of retinal, optic nerve and some central pathway function. A bright pen torch or Finhoff transilluminator is required. The light is shone into one eye and a normal response is seen as the pupil rapidly constricts (Fig. 3.8). This is the direct reflex. The opposite eye is examined (with the light still shining in the first eye) and constriction of the fellow pupil should occur—this is the consensual or indirect reflex. The light should then be moved to the second eye which is tested in the same way. The afferent nerve involved is the optic nerve (cranial nerve II), while the pupillary constriction is mediated by the parasympathetic fibres running in the oculomotor nerve (cranial nerve III).

The light source is then alternated between the two eyes in the swinging flashlight test. The light is shone into the first eye for a couple of seconds and then rapidly moved across to the second eye. A note is made of the response of the second pupil—it could constrict further, stay the same or dilate. A normal response would show both pupils staying miotic, often with further direct constriction of the newly illuminated pupil. If the second pupil suddenly dilates under direct illumination this is an abnormal response (called a positive swinging flashlight test) and indicates a lesion in the retina or optic nerve in this eye.

In addition to examining for the ability to constrict (it is abnormal for the pupil not to constrict), the speed and degree of constriction should also be evaluated. Animals which are very excited or aggressive will have slow and incomplete pupillary constriction as a result of increased sympathetic tone (adrenaline rush). Additionally, the resting position of both pupils should be assessed. They should be symmetrical and semi-dilated in dim light, with moderate constriction in room light.

Examination of the adnexa and anterior segment

Once vision has been assessed and the neurological testing performed, the systematic examination of the adnexa and anterior segment should be performed. Use of a pen torch will assist this general overview. Magnification can be helpful if available. If only one eye is affected, it is sensible to examine the normal eye first. A brief but through examination of eyelids, third eyelid, nasolacrimal punctae, conjunctiva, sclera, cornea, anterior chamber, iris and lens is performed. This examination is performed both in light and dark conditions. Ideally, a slit lamp biomicroscope should be used which gives excellent illumination and magnification (Table 3.4 and Fig. 3.9). However, these instruments are very costly, and so a combination of magnifying binocular loupes and a good direct light source can be employed. A direct ophthalmoscope can also be used. Settings of +20 are best for the lids and cornea, while +8 to +12 lenses are selected to examine the lens (direct ophthalmoscopy is mentioned in more detail later).

The eyelids are examined for position, the presence of swellings, eyelash abnormalities and the position and size of nasolacrimal punctae. The third eyelid is checked for colour, position, prolapse of the nictitans gland and abnormalities of cartilage. The conjunctival surfaces are examined for colour, swelling (chemosis), haemorrhage, moisture, masses and foreign bodies. The cornea is checked for transparency, vascularity, cellular infiltration, ulceration and alterations in shape. The anterior chamber is normally optically clear. In the presence of inflammation (uveitis), there will be leakage of proteins and cells, including sometimes

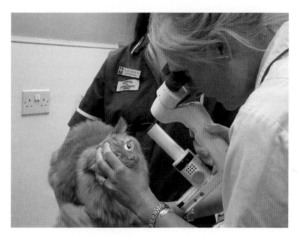

Fig. 3.9 Slit lamp examination.

red blood cells into the anterior chamber. This makes the aqueous cloudy and is termed aqueous flare. Frank blood in the anterior chamber is called hyphaema, while an abundant accumulation of white cells is termed hypopyon (and often looks like pus in the anterior chamber, although usually hypopyon is sterile). The anterior chamber is also assessed for depth. It might be deeper than normal if the lens is luxated into the posterior segment, or shallow if there are adhesions between the iris and the cornea (anterior synechia). Colour, adhesions, masses and persistent pupillary membrane remnants should be considered on iris examination. The lens is examined for optical clarity. The presence of an opacity in the lens is a cataract. Slit lamp biomicroscopy is invaluable in locating the site of cataract (e.g. posterior subcapsular, nuclear and so on). Examination of the lens is best performed once the pupil has been dilated.

Table 3.4 Advantages and disadvantages of the slit-lamp biomicroscope

Advantages	Disadvantages
<ul><li>High magnification (usually 10× to 16× for hand held types, more if table-mounted)</li><li>Full beam provides focussed illumination</li><li>Slit beam of variable widths</li><li>Photographic attachments available for some instruments (e.g. table-mounted slit-lamps)</li></ul>	<ul><li>Expensive</li><li>Learning curve for proper use</li><li>Can be cumbersome (especially table-mounted varieties)</li></ul>

Ophthalmoscopy

Both direct and indirect ophthalmoscopes can be used to examine the eye. The former are more common in general practice, although most ophthalmologists favour the latter! A summary of the advantages and disadvantages of the two methods is provided in Table 3.5.

Distant direct ophthalmoscopy

This technique is used to examine the eye for a clear visual axis and to assess pupil symmetry. It should be performed in the dark. A setting of 0 is used and the instrument is held to the examiner's eye at arm's length from the dog or cat (Fig. 3.10). The shine from reflective fundus is obtained (the glow from the tapetum seen through the pupil, called the fundic reflex). Any opacity in the visual axis will block the fundic reflex either totally or partially. This will be seen as a dark shadow within the bright fundic reflex. Opacities can be on the cornea, in the aqueous, lens or vitreous. By moving from side to side, one can assess the depth of the opacity. For example, a cataract on the anterior lens capsule will not move as you move your head because it is in the same plane as the pupil. A corneal opacity, which is in front of the plane of the pupil, will move in the same direction as you, while a cataract at the back of the lens, behind the pupil, will move away. This uses the phenomenon of parallax.

Distant direct ophthalmoscopy is also used to assess pupil size. Anisocoria (a difference in size between the two pupils) is detected more easily using this technique than by looking with the

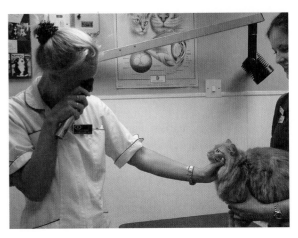

Fig. 3.10 Distant direct ophthalmoscopy.

naked eye. The observer looks through the instrument and, while light from the ophthalmoscope is shone from one eye to the other, compares the size of pupils.

Another useful aspect of distant direct ophthalmoscopy is that it can differentiate between a true cataract and the ageing change of nuclear sclerosis. Since a cataract is an opacity in the lens, it will appear as a dark shadow against the tapetal or fundic reflex as mentioned above. However, nuclear sclerosis is an age-related hardening of the lens. Although the condition renders the lens cloudy when viewed in the reflected light of a room, the direct light of the ophthalmoscope will pass right through it, with just a circular ring visible at the junction of the lens nucleus and cortex. Many owners, and some veterinary surgeons, mistakenly think a dog has cataracts when the diagnosis is nuclear sclerosis. If the method of distant direct ophthalmoscopy were used more

Table 3.5 A comparison of indirect and direct ophthalmoscopy		
	Indirect	**Direct**
Advantages	• Large field of view • Stereopsis • Can be used in semi-opaque media	• Easy to master • Cheap • High magnification • Upright image
Disadvantages	• Expensive • Inverted back to front image • Low magnification	• Small field of view • Very close to animal's teeth

frequently, owners would be saved the expense and time involved in referral to a specialist veterinary ophthalmologist only to be told that their pet has normal eyes for an older dog!

Complete examination of the lens, vitreous and fundus can only be achieved following mydriasis (pupil dilation). One drop of tropicamide 1.0% (Mydriacyl, Alcon) is applied to each eye. After 15–20 minutes the pupil should be fully dilated, allowing examination of the intraocular structures.

Close direct ophthalmoscopy

Examination of the adnexa and cornea was mentioned above. If a slit lamp biomicroscope is not available, examination of this part of the eye can still be readily achieved using a direct ophthalmoscope on a setting of +20 dioptres. The lens can be examined, after pupil dilation, using a setting of +8 to +12 dioptres.

To examine the fundus, a setting of 0 is chosen. If the observer has any known refractive errors (e.g. short sightedness) it will be necessary to adjust this setting in order to have a focussed image of the retina. One needs to be close to the patient—only 2–3 cm away from the eye (Fig. 3.11). Think of looking through a keyhole (the pupil)—the closer you are the more you will be able to see! It is sensible to start examining with the light on the ophthalmoscope quite dim, so that the animal gets used to your presence, before gradually increasing the rheostat brightness. This will be more comfortable for the patient, rather than diving straight in with the light on full brightness! Resting one finger on the bridge of the animal's nose will assist stabilisation and alert the observer to any change in position of the animal.

It is important to be systematic when examining the retina. First locate the optic disc. It is examined for colour, size and appearance of the blood vessels. The retina is then examined section by section. This is more challenging than in human ophthalmology as we cannot ask the patient to look up or to the right. However, with practice it becomes second nature and is most easily done by mentally splitting the back of the eye into quarters, starting from the optic disc and examining each quarter in turn. If you get disoriented by eye movement of the patient, finding the optic disc again will allow you to continue the systematic examination. It is important to look right out to the periphery, although this can be difficult laterally in dogs with long noses. It is often recommended to use the right eye when examining the patient's right eye, and left eye when examining the left. This is not essential providing the whole of the fundus is evaluated. By adding positive dioptre lenses in the ophthalmoscope it is possible to examine the vitreous.

Indirect ophthalmoscopy

This technique has advantages over direct ophthalmoscopy in that a large field of view is obtained, allowing a quick overview of the fundus. Binocular indirect ophthalmoscopy allows an appreciation of the fundus in 3-dimensions (therefore depressions and raised areas are more easily imaged). Indirect ophthalmoscopy also provides an improved image through opaque corneas and lenses. However, the image is inverted and back-to-front, and the magnification is less than with direct ophthalmoscopy. Ideally, both techniques should be employed.

A condensing lens is required (usually 20D, although pan retinal lenses offer a wider field of view (at greater cost!)). Monocular indirect ophthalmoscopy uses a bright light source (e.g. Finhoff transilluminator) held at the examiner's ear, while

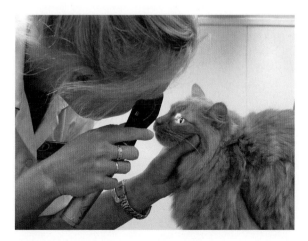

Fig. 3.11 Close direct ophthalmoscopy.

binocular indirect ophthalmoscopy utilises a special head or spectacle-mounted light source (Fig. 3.12). The examiner shines the light into the dilated pupil from approximately 50 cm away. Once the tapetal reflex is obtained, the condensing lens is moved into the line of vision just in front of the animal's eye. An upside down and back-to-front image of the fundus is obtained. However, with practice, our brains easily flip it the right way round for us to interpret. It is often necessary to move both the position and the angle of the lens to achieve the best image. This technique is more difficult to master than direct ophthalmoscopy but is certainly the preferred method of fundus examination among ophthalmologists. In addition, a teaching mirror can be fitted to most indirect headsets, allowing observers to view the same image as the ophthalmologist.

FURTHER EXAMINATION TECHNIQUES

Ophthalmic dyes

Fluorescein is an orange-coloured, water-soluble dye which stains corneal ulcers green. The intact cornea is lipophilic and, as such, does not allow uptake of fluorescein. However, once the epithelium is broken, the dye will adhere to the exposed stroma (which is hydrophilic). Impregnated strips (Fluorets, Chauvin) or single-use vials (Minims Fluorescein, Chauvin) can be used. If the strips are used, they should be moistened with sterile saline before being lightly touched onto the conjunctival surface (Fig. 3.13). Alternatively, a drop can be allowed to fall into the eye, as is done with the single-use vial. Multi-use preparations should be avoided as they are easily contaminated by potentially pathogenic bacteria. It is important to flush away excess dye with sterile saline to prevent false positives (e.g. irregularity of the corneal surface will allow pooling of the dye). Although corneal ulcers with exposed stroma will stain bright green, very deep ulcers might not; Descemet's membrane, the innermost layer of the cornea, does not take up the dye (because it is lipid-rich like the epithelium). Thus, if a pattern of staining around the edge but with a clear centre is observed, this is likely to be a very deep ulcer and is potentially extremely serious. Fluorescein can be safely used even in ruptured ulcers or corneal perforations as sterile fluorescein does not harm intraocular contents. Sometimes if the cornea has been perforated, a small stream of clear aqueous can be seen flowing through the fluorescein on the cornea (called a Seidel test). Staining is enhanced under blue and ultraviolet light (e.g. Wood's lamp) and because the results are immediate and obvious, it is always useful to demonstrate ulcers to owners. It helps them to understand the nature of their pet's problem much more easily.

A second corneal dye, rose Bengal, is sometimes used, mainly to detect ulcers due to herpes virus (FHV-1) in cats. It stains dead and devitalised epithelium a bright magenta colour and is

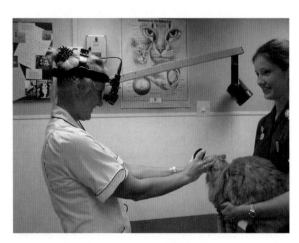

Fig. 3.12 Binocular indirect ophthalmoscopy.

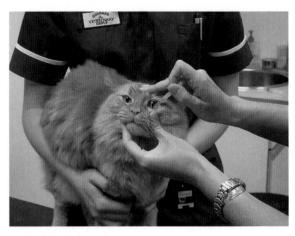

Fig. 3.13 Fluorescein dye.

more sensitive than fluorescein for the fine epithelial defects seen in herpetic keratitis. However, it is more irritant than fluorescein. In addition to flushing excess dye away before interpreting the results of the test, it is sensible to flush again at the end of the ophthalmic examination so that the patient is less likely to rub due to discomfort.

Nasolacrimal duct investigation

Initial assessment of the nasolacrimal drainage system can be made using fluorescein dye. A drop is placed in each eye and the nostrils are observed for the appearance of the bright green colour. Although the dye usually appears quickly, it can take up to 5 minutes. If no colour is seen, the mouth should be checked, since sometimes the nasolacrimal ducts have openings in the mouth (especially in brachycephalic breeds, in both dogs and cats). This test is quite unreliable and false negatives are common. For this reason, nasolacrimal flushing is often performed.

Under topical anaesthesia it is possible to cannulate the nasolacrimal punctae in dogs and rabbits, although cats often need sedation (Fig. 3.14). The ducts are assessed for patency using sterile saline solution, and this is more accurate than the fluorescein test mentioned above. Pliable plastic cannulae are recommended over metal ones in con-

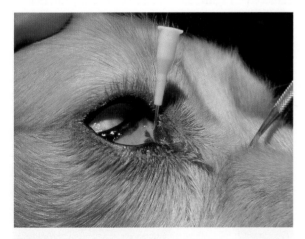

Fig. 3.14 Cannulation of the nasolacrimal punctum (upper one) prior to flushing to check patency of the nasolacrimal duct.

scious animals. It is easier to cannulate the upper punctum in cats and dogs (but rabbits only have one large lower punctum). A Nettleship's dilator, a pencil-like metal or plastic instrument, can be used to help to locate the punctae. In a normal patient, gentle flushing through the upper punctum, using sterile saline in a 5 ml syringe, will result in saline flowing through the lower punctum. This can be occluded with a finger, and saline will drip from the nose as the syringe is gently depressed. Some dogs will swallow as the solution drains into the mouth as well. The procedure is then repeated with the lower punctum cannulated. Saline is initially allowed to flow through the upper punctum before occluding this and allowing the solution to drain down to the nasal ostium. If there is a blockage, further investigation (including radiography) might be indicated; this is discussed later. Samples of the flushed material can be collected for bacterial (or occasionally fungal) culture and sensitivity.

Tonometry

Tonometry is the measurement of intraocular pressure (IOP). Normal intraocular pressure in dogs and cats is 10–25 mmHg. IOP can vary according to several factors, including breed (often higher in terriers), age (reduces with ageing) and the degree of restraint needed to measure the pressure (holding tightly around the neck will compress the jugular veins and could result in falsely elevated readings). Glaucoma is present if the intraocular pressure is clinically raised. Intraocular inflammation (i.e. uveitis) causes the pressure to drop below normal.

The instrument used to measure intraocular pressure is called a tonometer. Different types are available, but the most common ones in general use are the Schiotz tonometer (which measures by indenting the cornea, or indentation tonometry) and the more expensive Tonopen (which measures by flattening the cornea, or applanation tonometry). To measure IOP, animals should be unsedated but topical anaesthesia should be instilled into the eyes. Readings should be taken from both eyes. With both types of instrument, minimal restraint is required.

To use a Schiotz tonometer, the examiner must ensure the patient's eyes are in the horizontal plane. This usually means pointing the nose up to the ceiling, but without putting too much pressure around the neck. The footplate of the tonometer is allowed to rest on the cornea, and the reading is taken from the scale. Several readings should be taken from each eye. A conversion chart comes with the instrument such that the reading on the scale can be converted to mmHg. The Schiotz tonometer should not be used in very painful eyes or those with deep ulcers which could rupture. It is accurate to use but cumbersome, and some patients resent it. After each use, the instrument should be dismantled and thoroughly cleaned.

The Tonopen is a more user-friendly instrument and can be readily used by trained nurses (Fig. 3.15). It should be calibrated prior to use each day; instructions are easy to follow and come with the instrument. A new tip-cover is used for each patient, and after the application of topical anaesthesia the tip of the Tonopen is held perpendicular to the cornea and gently touched against it. The machine makes a beeping noise each time the cornea is touched, and after 3–5 touches a different beep is heard and the pressure appears as a digital reading in mmHg. The small screen also records the degree of error in the reading (this should be less than 5%). If it is higher than this, the reading is not accurate and the pressure should be measured again. The Tonopen is small and light to use, and the cornea does not need to be horizontal for measurements.

This means that the patient can have their head in a normal position, thus making them less resentful to the procedure. It can also be used in very small patients, such as kittens or rodents, as well as horses and farm animals. As with the Schiotz tonometer, care must be exercised with deep ulcers or corneal lacerations.

Another type of tonometer has recently been introduced into the veterinary market. The TonoVet tonometer is a rebound tonometer which seems to be easy to use and accurate. It is likely to become more popular in the near future.

Gonioscopy

Gonioscopy is the examination of the iridocorneal (drainage) angle. It is not possible to see the iridocorneal angle in dogs without the use of special contact lenses (goniolenses). Various different types of lenses are available, and personal preference usually dictates the type chosen. Koeppe and Barkan lenses are the most frequently encountered. These are placed on the anaesthetised cornea and allow the light to be bent (refracted) such that the drainage angle can be evaluated (Fig. 3.16). The lenses basically allow the ophthalmologist to look around the corner, between the cornea and the iris. The technique is used mainly in dogs to check for abnormalities in this angle (goniodysgenesis) which predispose to the development of primary glaucoma. Figure 3.17 illustrates the appearance of

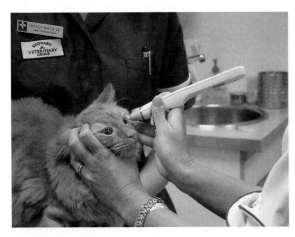

Fig. 3.15 Tonometry using a Tonopen.

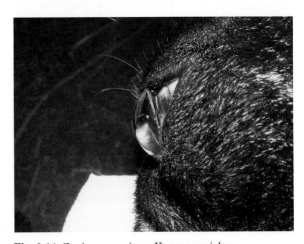

Fig. 3.16 Gonioscopy using a Koeppe goniolens.

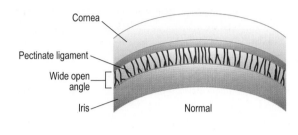

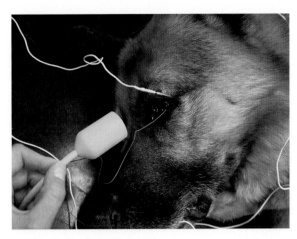

Fig. 3.18 Electroretinography.

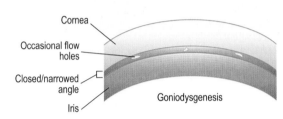

Fig. 3.17 Gonioscopic appearance of a normal drainage angle and one affected with goniodysgenesis.

a normal drainage angle and one affected by goniodysgenesis. If one eye is glaucomatous, the fellow eye is examined for evidence of goniodysgenesis. Gonioscopy is also used to screen dogs for goniodysgenesis in breeds known to suffer from primary inherited glaucoma, e.g. Bassett hounds, flat coated retrievers and Welsh springer spaniels, among others.

Electroretinography

The electroretinogram (ERG) is the electrical response recorded when the retina is stimulated with light. It is not a measure of vision (the ERG will be normal in central blindness) but measures the integrity of the outer retinal layers, including the retinal pigment epithelium. It is used mainly to establish retinal function when opacification (usually cataract) prevents visualisation of the fundus. In this situation it is very important to establish that the retina is working normally if cataract surgery is being considered. Inherited retinal degenerations are common in pedigree dogs, and cataracts frequently develop along with the degeneration. Cataract surgery would not restore vision if the retina is atrophied, which is why the test is so important. ERGs are also used to investigate

cases of sudden blindness where the eye looks normal, in order to differentiate sudden acquired retinal degeneration (SARD) from optic neuritis or central blindness.

Patients are usually lightly sedated to perform an ERG, although in some animals general anaesthesia is preferred. A special contact lens electrode filled with a viscous gel (such as 2% hypromellose or carbomer 980) is placed on the cornea, while ground and reference needle electrodes are placed subcutaneously, usually at the nuchal crest and lateral canthus, respectively (Fig. 3.18). These are connected to a computer system and light source. Animals usually need to spend about 20 minutes in the dark (called dark adaptation) prior to ERG testing so that the retina is maximally sensitive to the stimulating light. Different protocols of light stimulation are used (single flashes of differing light intensity, flickers of light and so on), which can stimulate rods and cones separately. The response of the retina is recorded graphically, and various measurements can be taken (e.g. the amplitude of the response). If no response is recorded this indicates no functional retina, as is found in end-stage progressive retinal atrophy and sudden acquired retinal degeneration (SARD).

Blood pressure measurement

The measurement of blood pressure is routinely performed in ophthalmic patients since hypertension is a common cause of ocular disease in both dogs and, especially, cats. Indirect measurement is routinely employed, and two main methods are available: the Doppler and oscillometric systems (Fig. 6.9).

Doppler blood pressure monitors usually only detect the systolic blood pressure and measure the flow of blood within an artery distal to the site of an inflatable cuff which is used to initially occlude the flow. The oscillometric method relies on the detection of the oscillations of pressure induced in an inflatable cuff by the pulsatile flow of blood though an artery beneath. This method allows the detection of both systolic and diastolic pressures, as well as mean arterial pressure. Both methods are reliable in dogs and anaesthetised cats, but unfortunately the oscillometric technique cannot be used in all cats. In a proportion of conscious cats no meaningful measurements can be detected and, for this reason, the Doppler system remains the preferred method of blood pressure detection in this species. The Doppler units are also significantly cheaper to buy!

To measure blood pressure accurately, several factors need to be considered. The patient should be as relaxed as possible and attempts must be made to minimise stress. The measurement should be taken in a quiet room with minimal other activity going on, and the patient should be given time to acclimatise to the surroundings (at least 10 minutes is recommended). Often patients are less stressed if owners are present, particularly nervous cats. Gentle and sympathetic handling is important since the stress of restraint can increase blood pressure significantly.

There are three main sites for measuring blood flow. The most commonly chosen is the forelimb (detecting blood flow in the common digital artery), but the hind limb (detecting flow in the cranial tibial artery) and the tail (detecting blood flow in the medial coccygeal artery) can also be employed.

For the Doppler method using the forelimb, a small area of fur can be clipped from behind the paw between the carpal and metacarpal pads, or this area must be thoroughly wetted with alcohol/surgical spirit to improve signal detection. A cuff of correct size is placed around the antebrachium below the elbow (Fig. 3.19) The cuff

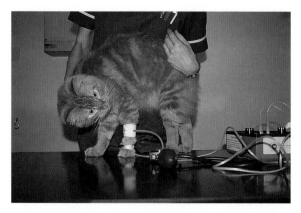

Fig. 3.19 Measurement of blood pressure using a Doppler machine.

width can affect blood pressure reading, and the most accurate width is 40% of the limb circumference in dogs and 30% limb circumference in cats. A standard 2.5 cm width is usually chosen for cats. Ultrasound coupling gel is applied to both the clipped area and to the Doppler probe which is then placed gently over the area of the artery, keeping the alignment of Doppler crystals perpendicular to the artery. The sound should be turned down very low until the signal is detected, since the noise from moving the probe can stress the patient. Alternatively, head phones can be worn. Once the pulsatile blood flow is heard, the probe can be taped in place. It is important to only use gentle pressure when locating the blood flow since it is easy to occlude the artery, especially in smaller patients.

Once regular pulsatile blood flow can be heard, the cuff is inflated to 30–40 mmHg above the point at which the blood flow can no longer be heard. The air is slowly allowed to bleed out from the valve, and the reading is taken when the sound of the blood flow can first be detected again. This is the systolic blood pressure. The measurement should be repeated until at least 5 consecutive readings of similar value are obtained, and these are then averaged. Often the first 2–3 readings taken are significantly higher (again due to stress), and these should not be included when calculating the average.

Oscillometric machines are simpler to use, providing a signal can be recorded. The transducer is located within the cuff, and once positioned the

Table 3.6 Normal blood pressure readings

Reading in mmHG	Dog	Cat	Man
Systolic	110–190	120–170	110–140
Diastolic	55–110	70–120	70–100

machine will automatically inflate and deflate the cuff to provide a digital readout of the systolic, diastolic and mean arterial pressures together with the heart rate. Several readings should be taken over a 5–10 minute period.

Normal blood pressure readings are listed in Table 3.6. In borderline cases where the readings obtained are 10–20 mmHg above the normal range, it is important to repeat the readings on several occasions, both on the same day and on subsequent visits, before deciding whether the readings are significantly elevated. Obviously, the clinical condition of the patient, together with any laboratory investigations, should be taken into consideration when reviewing the measurements obtained.

LABORATORY INVESTIGATION

The collection and handling of samples from the eyes is commonly performed in veterinary ophthalmology. Samples collected include swabs, scrapings and other samples for cytology, aspirates and biopsy specimens. They are useful for the investigation of suspected infectious disease, as well as immune-mediated and neoplastic processes.

Swabs

Swabs can be taken from the conjunctiva, cornea or discharges. It is important to tell the laboratory exactly where the sample has been taken from. A sterile swab is gently rolled across the appropriate surface. A topical anaesthesia is not usually required (it can affect interpretation of the results and can have a bacteriostatic effect which is not desirable when trying to isolate such pathogens). If the sample is for cytology, then a dry swab is used and cellular integrity is usually preserved (but there are better methods of sample collection for cytology; see below). The majority of swabs

taken are for microbial analysis, and in this instance it is better to use a moistened swab (either with sterile saline, or the appropriate culture medium). This gives a better yield of pathogens. It is important not to touch the swab against other parts of the eye since it could become contaminated with bacteria which are normally present on the ocular surface.

Swabs should be labelled and dated prior to being dispatched. Previous and current medication should be detailed since this can affect interpretation of the results. If there is any delay between sample collection and processing then the swab should be refrigerated (but not frozen). The culture requirements for bacteria, *Chlamydophila*, *Mycoplasma*, fungi and viruses can all vary, and if there is any uncertainty about the best media for collection, it is important to discuss this with the laboratory. In addition to culture, the sample should undergo sensitivity testing by suitable antimicrobials.

Swabs taken for viral culture (or virus isolation) are usually for feline herpes virus (FHV-1), and special culture media are required. Combined media for FHV-1 and *Chlamydophila* are routinely used. Swabs are usually obtained both from the conjunctiva and the oropharynx. These samples can be frozen if there is any delay in dispatch to the laboratory (over the weekend for example), but it is always sensible to check this with the laboratory first.

Scrapings and other samples for cytology

Scrapings are usually used for cytological examination. They are useful mainly for inflammatory and neoplastic conditions, but are of use in the investigation of infectious processes as well. Samples can be taken from eyelids in exactly the same way as from other skin sites. A scalpel blade is used and the tissue gently squeezed during the scraping to express material from the glands and hair follicles. It is important that the eyelid margins are not damaged, and since the procedure can result in some swelling and discomfort afterwards, the animal must be monitored to prevent self-trauma. Scrapings from the conjunctiva and cornea require topical anaesthesia and sometimes sedation of the patient. Holding a sterile cotton bud moistened with topical anaesthesia against the area to be sampled for 30–60 seconds will achieve a deeper numbing than a single drop of anaesthetic. A specialised instrument is available for scraping the cornea and conjunctiva—the Kimura spatula. However, most people use the blunt end of a scalpel blade for convenience (Fig. 3.20). The material obtained is gently spread across a dry microscope slide.

Another way of collecting samples for cytology is to use a cytobrush. These are small nylon-bristled brushes that look like mascara-wands. They were initially designed for gynaecological use but are popular for ocular cytology since they are safe to use and maintain good cellular integrity, as well as distributing the cells evenly. Once the material is collected by gently rolling the brush over the surface of the tissue, it is then rolled again over a dry microscope slide.

A final technique for sample collection for cytology is the impression smear, which is also very easy to perform. A dry microscope slide is pressed firmly against the tissue to be sampled, and any cells which readily exfoliate are transferred to the slide.

Whichever method of sample collection is used, the principles for processing the specimens are the same. Samples are gently spread on a clean microscope slide and air-dried. In-house assessment using Diff-quik stains and Gram stains can be useful for bacterial identification, the presence of fungi and the evaluation of cell types, but samples should also be sent to a cytologist for professional interpretation. It is useful to send unstained samples as well, since further specialist stains can be used if indicated (e.g. immunofluorescence stains for feline herpes virus and *Chlamydophila*).

Aspirates

Aspirates can be taken from ocular tissue in the same way as sampling from elsewhere in the body. They are useful for investigating masses involving the adnexa, orbit or the eye itself. Abscesses, granulomas, tumours (such as lymphomas and mast cell tumours) and cysts can be differentiated. Inadvertent globe damage can be avoided by making sure that the animal is suitably restrained (with light sedation if necessary) and always directing the needle away from the globe. The area to be sampled is stabilised if possible, and the needle is inserted without the syringe attached. Suction is then applied, and the needle is redirected several times to get a representative sample. The syringe is removed, filled with air and then reconnected to the needle. The sample obtained is then expressed onto a microscope slide. A second slide is used to gently spread the material. Occasionally, it is necessary to centrifuge the sample prior to smear preparation if cellular yield is likely to be low (e.g. samples taken from the anterior chamber). In addition to cytology, microbial analysis can be performed on aspirates by placing the material on a moistened swab as detailed above.

It is sometimes helpful to perform imaging techniques, such as radiography and ultrasonography, prior to sample collection, and ultrasound-guided biopsy is beneficial for retrobulbar lesions. General anaesthesia is usually required for these, and the approach to the retrobulbar space can be lateral, transconjunctival or oral. Intraocular aspirates are occasionally taken by specialists using general anaesthesia, often with the assistance of an

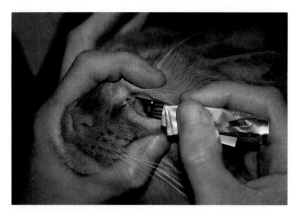

Fig. 3.20 Scrapes for cytology.

operating microscope for magnification. Such procedures carry significant risks (e.g. intraocular haemorrhage, lens rupture and retinal detachment) and are discussed further in Chapter 8.

Biopsy and complete histological examination

Biopsy samples can be taken where the pathological process is too deep for scrapes and smears to be of use, or when the actual architecture of the tissues, rather than just the cells involved, needs to be examined. Samples should be placed in their correct orientation on card before putting in the fixative to make interpretation easier. If necessary, samples can be sent for microbial investigation as well as histology.

Conjunctival biopsies are taken after the area has been desensitised with a cotton bud soaked in topical anaesthetic, as mentioned above. An area of conjunctiva is tented up, using a fine pair of rat-toothed forceps, and a piece is snipped off from below using small sharp scissors. No sutures are needed, as the area heals rapidly. Some haemorrhage can be expected but soon stops if gentle pressure is applied.

Eyelid biopsies are taken under general anaesthesia if wedge-sections including the eyelid margin are needed. Sometimes, punch biopsies can be taken with the animal sedated. Histology can be performed on biopsy samples from the cornea, and these are obtained by surgical keratectomy under general anaesthesia.

A complete histological examination is frequently performed on enucleated globes. Examples include painful blind eyes due to refractive uveitis or hyphaema, glaucoma or endophthalmitis. Histology can help to understand the pathologic processes which lead to loss of the eye and can be useful for ongoing case management (e.g. typing tumours). Correct handling of the specimen is required prior to submission to the laboratory. All tissue apart from the optic nerve should be trimmed from the globe— the histopathologist does not require eyelids and muscle if the pathology is contained within the eye. If there are concerns about the periocular tissues (e.g. tumour spread), these can be submitted separately if nec-

essary; leaving them on the enucleated globe will only reduce penetration of the fixative. Most globes will be fixed in formalin, but several specialist media are available and consultation with the pathologist might be useful. All fixatives are potentially dangerous, and due attention to health and safety issues must be paid in handling them. It is important to give the pathologist as much information as possible. In addition to the animal's details and which eye is submitted, information about the clinician's findings should be included. A copy of their ophthalmic examination report together with diagrams of any focal lesions will be of great assistance. Details of any medical or surgical treatments plus any findings in the fellow eye should be submitted.

Other laboratory investigations

Other laboratory investigations include polymerase chain reactions (PCR) and serology. PCR technology has advanced in recent years and provides an extremely sensitive and specific test for microbial detection. It relies on the identification of a section of DNA from the organism in question, and samples containing more DNA, such as biopsies, are more likely to yield positive results than smears or swabs. However, since the technique is so sensitive, it can identify minute quantities of DNA and care must be exercised in interpretation, particularly for diseases in which a carrier status exists (e.g. FHV-1). Just because a pathological organism is identified, this does not necessarily mean that it is causing the disease.

Serology assesses the animal's response to an organism. It shows whether an animal has been exposed to the organism (through infection or vaccination) but does not correlate this with the clinical disease. For example, over 95% of cats show serological evidence of exposure to FHV-1, but the antibody reaction does not mean that they are currently actively infected with the virus. Paired samples taken 1–2 weeks apart which show a rising titre might be indicative of active infection and are more useful than a single test.

Genetic assessment is becoming available for some inherited ocular diseases, and samples of the animal's DNA (usually blood or buccal mucosa) can be analysed to test for some specific genetic diseases (e.g. progressive retinal atrophy in the Irish setter, Cardigan Welsh corgi and miniature schnauzer). Hopefully, these techniques will become more widely available in future as the specific gene mutations causing the diseases are identified, enabling tests to be developed to detect them.

OCULAR IMAGING

Various imaging techniques are available for examining the eye, orbit and central pathways. If the structures of the eye cannot be directly visualised (due to corneal opacification, hyphaema or cataract, for example) clinicians resort to imaging techniques such as ultrasonography. Radiography is useful for some types of orbital disease (e.g. fractures), while more sophisticated techniques for central imaging include magnetic resonance imaging and computed tomography. Often, more than one technique is employed to gain as much information about the disease process as possible.

Radiography

Plain and contrast X-rays of the head are very useful for some ocular and orbital diseases. Radiography is relatively cheap and available to all. However, disadvantages include interpretation of this complex area, the use of ionising radiation and poor soft tissue differentiation.

The skull is complex, with both intra- and inter-species variations. A good knowledge of anatomy is needed before an understanding of the normal radiographic appearance can be obtained. It is useful to have a skull to manipulate to understand the relationship between the different bones, teeth, air pockets within sinuses and so on, as well as reference books to consult. Radiography is used to investigate retrobulbar lesions, suspected foreign bodies (which only show up if radiopaque) and to examine for evidence of bony lysis, usually associated with neoplasia. Dental disease can cause ocular signs, and careful examination of the maxillary dental arcade is important. If only soft tissue involvement is present in the disease, X-rays are less useful. The placing of a

radiopaque marker at the eyes will assist with interpretation. Circular wires (Fleiringa rings) can be positioned over one or both eyes since the globes themselves are not visible on X-ray.

Careful positioning is mandatory. If neoplasia is suspected, intra-oral views should be taken in addition to routine dorsoventral and lateral views. Open mouth rostrocaudal views can also be helpful for retrobulbar investigation and if nasal or tympanic bullae involvement is suspected (Fig. 3.21 a, b & c). General anaesthesia is clearly required for these. For intra-oral views, high-definition film is needed and should be placed as far back into the mouth as possible.

Radiography of the chest and abdomen should be performed if neoplastic disease is suspected. Many retrobulbar tumours are malignant, with the potential for metastasis. Some fungal diseases can be disseminated, and radiography of the chest in particular might be helpful.

Contrast radiography

This is used to delineate space-occupying lesions, locate foreign bodies and identify blockages. Dacryocystorhinography is the use of contrast material to outline the nasolacrimal system and is employed to assess patency and to locate blockages. It is used in the investigation of epiphora and ocular discharge. Plain X-rays are taken under general anaesthesia, and then the upper nasolacrimal punctum is cannulated and the lower one occluded. A small amount (approximately 2 ml) of water-soluble iodinated contrast material is gently injected, and lateral and dorsoventral views are repeated. Although both left and right can be injected with contrast to compare the pathways of the ducts, lateral views are confused and difficult to interpret if this is done. Normally, it is sufficient to examine only the affected side. Dacryocystorhinography is useful in rabbits, as tooth problems affecting both the incisors and molars can lead to dacryocystitis (inflammation of the nasolacrinial duct). The rabbit only has a lower nasolacrimal punctum, and a small amount of contrast material is sufficient: 0.2–0.5 ml.

Other contrast techniques are rarely used. Orbital venograms are useful if vascular abnor-

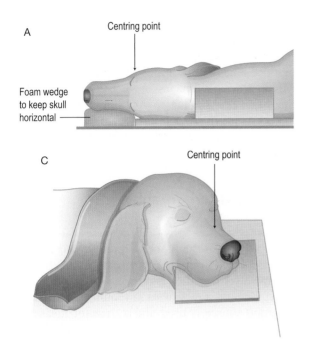

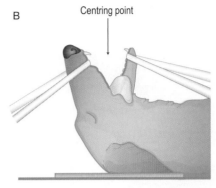

Fig. 3.21 Positioning of the head for skull radiography: a) lateral skull; b) intra-oral positioning; c) open mouth rostrocaudal view.

malities, such as arteriovenous shunts, are suspected. Contrast sialography (injection of contrast material into the salivary glands) can be used to investigate suspected sialocoeles. However, other imaging techniques have largely superseded these methods.

Ultrasonography

Ocular and orbital ultrasonography revolutionised things back in the late 1970s and early 1980s. It is a non-invasive, non-harmful procedure which can usually be performed in conscious or lightly sedated animals. As such, it has largely replaced radiography as a first line of ophthalmic diagnostic imaging. Anatomical images of ocular contents are obtained when it is not possible to examine them directly due to opacification from cataract or corneal oedema, for example. It can be used to measure ocular distances, evaluate the extent of tumours (both within the eye and in the periocular region) and to visualise retrobulbar structures. Two main types of ultrasound examination are available:

- **A mode** (amplitude mode) provides a 1-dimensional acoustic display which is used

almost exclusively for measurement (e.g. to determine microphthalmos or to compare anterior chamber depth).
- **B mode** (brightness mode) is the most useful in practice. A 7.5–10.0 MHz sector transducer is used, although higher frequency (12.5, 15 and 20 MHz) will provide greater resolution but less depth of imaging. Higher frequency probes give better resolution of the anterior chamber and lens, for example, but are not suitable for retrobulbar investigation. Small, portable units especially designed for veterinary ophthalmology are becoming available.

After the application topical anaesthesia and water-based ultrasound gel, the eye can be scanned. Occasionally, sedation is required but most dogs and cats accept the procedure quite readily. Both horizontal and vertical planes should be imaged. A stand off is advisable if anterior segment detail is examined (without one it is not possible to examine the cornea, and detail of the anterior chamber is lost as well). Some transducers have these built in, but a water- or gel-filled glove is an acceptable alternative. Direct transcorneal scanning offers better resolution than through the lids since trapped air in the latter creates artefacts (Fig. 3.22). A temporal approach

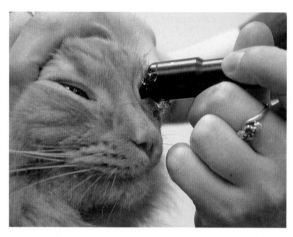

Fig. 3.22 Performing ultrasonography.

is useful to visualise retrobulbar structures, including the optic nerve.

Often we are lucky and have a normal and abnormal eye, and it is useful to scan both and compare images. It is possible to detect a whole range of abnormalities using B Mode ultrasonography, including retrobulbar tumours, abscesses and foreign bodies, intraocular tumours, retinal detachments, lens luxations, persistent hyaloid vessels and ocular ruptures. Ultrasound-guided biopsies can be taken of retrobulbar lesions to obtain specimens for analysis.

Colour Doppler imaging (CDI) is becoming more widely used and provides simultaneous imaging of ocular structures with real time B mode ultrasonography, with superimposed colour-coded Doppler evaluation of vascular velocity patterns. It is non-invasive, but animals often need to be anaesthetised or heavily sedated since the procedure takes longer than ultrasonography alone. Arteries pulsate while veins have continuous flow. Blood flow towards the transducer is red while that away from it is blue. There is a wide variability in the vascular patterns between various breeds, making interpretation difficult, although as previously mentioned, we can usually compare the diseased eye with the normal fellow eye. Indications for the use of colour Doppler imaging include cases of head trauma, acute glaucoma and cellulitis (where a reduction in the vascular pattern has been seen), ciliary body melanoma (where neovascularisation has been described) and arteriovenous shunts.

High-frequency ultrasound biomicroscopy is also becoming available, although the cost of the machines makes it unlikely to be seen in private practice. The use of very high frequencies (50–100 MHz) produces images of such high resolution that they are similar to low-power microscopy images. This is useful for examination of the drainage angle, the depth of corneal sequestra in cats and the extent of iridal tumours, for example.

Computed tomography

Computed tomography (CT) provides a 2-dimensional section of the tissue of interest, and images are digitised through a computer which can manipulate them into 3-dimensional representations. General anaesthesia is required. A rotating radiation source is used and a detector measures the attenuation of the beam through the subject. On the image obtained, areas which absorb more X-rays are light grey while darker areas are seen with less absorbing tissues, just as in conventional X-rays. For example, fat is seen as black with a low density of absorption while the optic nerves are dense and bright white. There is a high contrast between orbital soft tissues and surrounding bone, and anatomical detail is good. The detail obtained of soft tissues is far better than with conventional X-rays, but not as good as that seen with magnetic resonance imaging. Further contrast enhancement can be obtained by the use of iodinated radiographic contrast agents.

Indications for CT include the investigation of orbital disease, including retrobulbar masses, orbital fractures and suspected foreign bodies (of any nature). It is the modality of choice following head or orbital trauma, such as seen in road traffic accidents.

Magnetic resonance imaging

Magnetic resonance imaging (MRI) relies on the proton density (hydrogen ion content) of tissues. The subject is placed in a strong magnetic field and nuclei with odd numbers of protons and neutrons become magnetised and line-up in the field. A smaller surface coil is positioned over the area to be

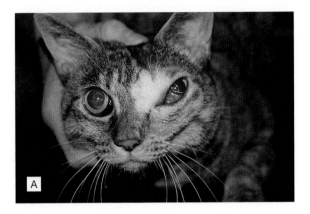

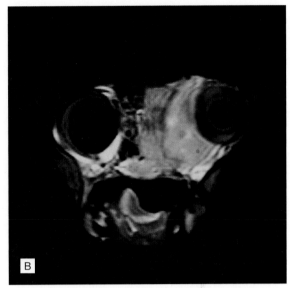

Fig. 3.23 a) clinical presentation of a cat with a retrobulbar mass; b) MRI image of the same cat showing extent of tumour in retrobulbar space and nasal chambers (sarcoma).

imaged, and radio waves are then applied which cause the tissues to resonate. Images are obtained which depend upon the physical and chemical properties of each tissue. Various different settings are used to highlight different tissue properties, and special contrast media can be injected to further highlight various tissues. Images take about 45 minutes to be obtained, and the patient must be completely still during this time—thus general anaesthesia is required. Special anaesthetic equipment might be required as no ferrous metals can be used since these will be affected by the magnetic field. For this reason the technique is not suitable if metallic foreign bodies are suspected; they could move in the magnetic field and cause serious damage to the eye or periocular tissues. Images can be obtained in different planes without the need to reposition the patient and, as such, excellent 3-dimensional images can be produced.

Indications for MRI are similar to CT, but it provides better soft tissue resolution and is the preferred imaging technique if optic nerve or intracranial lesions (e.g. tumour over the optic chiasm) are suspected. Retrobulbar disease, such as cellulitis or tumours, can be clearly delineated (Fig. 3.23), but CT offers better detail if bony involvement is suspected. In addition, intraocular disease (such as uveal masses and retinal detachments) can be readily identified. However, it is not usually necessary to resort to MRI as a diagnostic tool for these, as ultrasonography is sufficient! Table 3.7 highlights the advantages and disadvantages of MRI and CT.

Table 3.7 Comparison of MRI and CT		
	MRI	**CT**
Advantages	• Non-ionising • Direct multiplanar images • No known side-effects • Good soft tissue resolution • Safe contrast agents	• Excellent bony detail • Safe with metal objects • Less costly • Relatively quick image collection
Disadvantages	• Expensive • Long data acquisition time • Cannot be used for ferrous foreign bodies	• Ionising radiation used • Patient repositioning necessary for multiple views

BIBLIOGRAPHY AND FURTHER READING

Grahn B, Cullen C, Peiffer R. Veterinary ophthalmology essentials. Oxford: Butterworth-Heinemann; 2004.

Petersen-Jones S, Crispin S, eds. BSAVA manual of small animal ophthalmology. 2nd edn. Gloucester: British Small Animal Veterinary Association; 2002.

Veterinary Technician 2004; January issue (focusing on ophthalmology).

4 Medical nursing for ophthalmic patients

INTRODUCTION

Many patients with eye diseases need to be hospitalised for various reasons and their nursing care can be critical to the successful outcome of their problems. In this chapter we will consider various aspects of medical ophthalmic nursing, starting when the patient is admitted to the practice and finishing when the patient is discharged. We will also discuss advice to owners, with special reference to looking after blind pets.

ADMITTANCE TO THE HOSPITAL

The owners will have had a consultation with the veterinary surgeon prior to the admission of their pet and should have some understanding of the reason for hospitalisation—cataract surgery or the intensive treatment of a melting corneal ulcer, for example. The admittance nurse should ask the owners if they have any further questions or concerns before their pet is admitted, as sometimes they are more likely to talk to the nurse than the ophthalmologist! They often have worries about where their pet will be kept and how often they will be checked overnight, for example. Showing the client the hospital facilities can also help allay their concerns.

There should be a consent form for the owner to sign (Fig. 6.2, p. 84). In addition to the owner information, this should provide details of the reason for admittance together with an idea of the costs involved. If the animal is admitted for surgery, the nurse must check when the animal last received food and water and whether preoperative blood tests are advised. Contact telephone numbers must be obtained, and if more than one number is provided it is sensible to get the owners to indicate which is likely to be the best number to try first. The nurse should check the animal's heart and respiratory rates on admittance, and record them on the consent form or hospital record sheet, so that there is a baseline for comparison later if needed. It is very important to establish whether the patient is receiving any medication at all, either for the eye problem or for an unrelated disease. For example, many patients for cataract surgery are older and may be on medication for arthritis or cardiac problems. If the patient is on medication, this must be noted, together with details of when the medication was

Table 4.1 Checklist for hospital admission
• Check owner and patient details are correct
• Reason for admittance
• Quote for procedure included
• Contact telephone numbers
• Record pulse and respiration rates (temperature if requested by clinician)
• Record visual status of patient
• Current medications—ocular and systemic
• Special diets
• Any personal belongings (collar, blanket, etc.)
• Any specific details—kennel guarder, will only urinate on grass, hates cats!

Table 4.2 Checklist for blind patients
• Talk to them—especially before handling
• Dogs on short lead
• Own bowl and bedding for familiarity
• Show them to the water bowl in kennel
• Choose kennel for easy access to outside
• Label on kennel door stating blind

last given and when the next dose is due. Many patients are on special diets, so again this should be checked. Once this information has been obtained, the owner should be asked to sign the consent form. This procedure is summarised in Table 4.1.

Another very important thing to establish before the animal is admitted is whether the patient can see. Remember that some ophthalmic patients will be blind and special attention is needed to their care. It can be a stressful experience for any dog or cat to be hospitalised, but imagine how disorienting it would be for the blind animal. Often having a blanket or toy from home will help these patients settle. It is worthwhile spending time in the consulting room with the owners and their pet, getting to know the animal before taking it into the hospital kennels. This will help the pet to feel more secure, having someone familiar looking after them, and will also reassure the owners. Sometimes having the owners come through to the kennels with their pet will be of benefit to the patient, depending on circumstances. Blind animals will need far more talking to and gentle reassurance than visual patients. If admitting a blind dog, it is important to keep it on a very short lead and guide it through the hospital. Smaller dogs can be carried if they are frightened and unwilling to walk. Once in the kennels, the patient should be made as comfortable as possible in the cage, and shown where its water and food bowls are. Many practices have notices to put on the kennel door (e.g. care, nil by mouth, sedated and so on), and it is useful to have one for blind patients. A checklist for blind patients is shown in Table 4.2. Further information about

care of the blind pet is included later in this chapter.

GENERAL IN-PATIENT CARE

An example in-patient record sheet is shown in Figure 4.1.

Choice of cages

Most hospital cages are stainless steel, with bars on the doors. Unfortunately, patients can rub against the bars and potentially damage the eyes. Glass-fronted cages might be more appropriate (Fig. 4.2). For the same reason, catches should be outside the cage where the animal cannot reach them. Cages should be large enough for the pet to move comfortably, with space for bowls and a litter tray if required.

Bedding

Familiar smells can help animals to settle in their cages and so bedding from home can be comforting. Obviously, owners must be made aware that bedding from home can get soiled and must be washable. Animals must be checked to see that they are not able to self-traumatise with the bedding (e.g. ruffling a blanket in the corner can allow a dog to rub its eyes against it, or cats might hide under their bedding and rub unobserved).

Food and water

As with all hospitalised patients, it is important to monitor food and water intake. Adequate nutrition is vital during recovery from disease of any sort, and ocular problems are no exception. For blind patients, remember that they might require assistance in finding water and food bowls. Ani-

mals should be tempted to eat—hand feeding, warming the food, offering odorous food and the animal's favourite titbits should be practised

INPATIENT RECORD

DATE		VET		
PATIENT	**OWNER**	**AGE**	**SEX**	**WEIGHT**

CONDITION

TODAY'S INSTRUCTIONS

DIET \ NUTRITION

FLUID THERAPY

OWNER SPOKEN TO   AM Yes / No initial ………   PM Yes / No initial ………
Comments

TREATMENT

DRUG	DOSE	ROUTE	FREQUENCY
DRUG	**DOSE**	**ROUTE**	**FREQUENCY**
DRUG	**DOSE**	**ROUTE**	**FREQUENCY**
DRUG	**DOSE**	**ROUTE**	**FREQUENCY**
DRUG	**DOSE**	**ROUTE**	**FREQUENCY**

Fig. 4.1 In-patient hospital record sheet.

DRUG	DOSE	ROUTE	FREQUENCY
DRUG	DOSE	ROUTE	FREQUENCY

INPATIENT OBSERVATIONS

TIME	T	P	R	E	D	U	F	OBSERVATIONS

Fig. 4.1 In-patient hospital record sheet—*continued*.

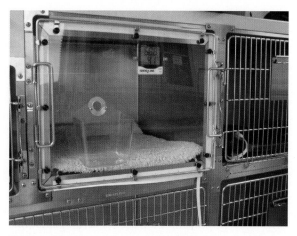

Fig. 4.2 Glass-fronted cage to prevent inadvertent damage to eyes.

routinely. As we would expect with good nursing practice, the same bowls should be used for the duration of the patient's hospital stay. Remember that blind patients are often clumsy, and stable bowls should be chosen to reduce the risk of accidental spillage. Sometimes the provision of familiar bowls from home will assist voluntary feeding.

Urination and defecation

Urination and defecation also need monitoring. For dogs, frequent trips to the outside run or grassy area should be undertaken, remembering that a short lead and constant talking-to are important in visually-impaired animals. Blind animals must never be left unattended in exercise areas. It is sensible to site such patients in kennels where there is easy access to outside areas, thus avoiding confusing routes for them. Patients with diabetes mellitus are frequently hospitalised for cataract surgery. Even if the diabetes mellitus is well-controlled, the patient might still be polyuric and will need to be given adequate opportunity to urinate. Blind cats should be put in their litter tray several times until they learn its location.

Cleansing and application of medicines

Most patients hospitalised with ocular problems will require topical medication and often systemic drugs. Each patient should have their own labelled medications; the use of multi-patient 'kennels' drops is to be discouraged. The frequency of administration will be determined by the veterinary surgeon. Ideally, the application of such drugs should be spread over 24 hours: three-times-daily medication should be given every 8 hours (e.g. 8 a.m., 4 p.m. and midnight); four-times-daily should be given every 6 hours (e.g. 8 a.m., 2 p.m., 8 p.m., 2 a.m.). Unfortunately, not all veterinary surgeries provide 24-hour nursing cover, and medications might need to be fitted in to the working day. In some situations, the patient might be better off at home where the owner can medicate more often!

A daily hospital sheet (Fig. 4.1) should be provided for each patient. Along with patient details and the reason for admission, this should include all medications the animal requires (including fluids if necessary) along with a space for observation (i.e. feeding, water intake, nature of ocular discharge, evidence of pain, etc.). Certain eye preparations need refrigeration, and it is important to note this on the record sheet. Otherwise, further bottles might be opened unnecessarily by a nurse on a later shift who cannot find the drops!

Before the application of topical medication, any ocular discharge should be gently removed. There is no point in applying medication to a dirty eye since the therapeutic effect might be reduced as the medication sits in mucus, for example. The nature and extent of any discharge should be recorded, and if it is excessive or different from that previously recorded, the clinician in charge of the case should be notified before cleansing. A moistened lint-free swab should be used to clean the eye, sweeping gently from medially to laterally. Use a second clean swab to wipe any discharge accumulated at the medial canthus or on the face. Obviously, a separate swab should be used for each eye. If the patient is on several topical preparations, the order of their application should be indicated by the clinician. In general, drops should always be applied before gels or ointments. At least 10 minutes should elapse between subsequent medications— the reasons for this are discussed in Chapter 2, along with details of exactly how to apply drops and ointments. A summary for topical application is listed in Table 4.3, while

Table 4.3 Application of topical medication

- Clean any discharge
- Gentle restraint
- Nose slightly elevated
- Come from behind the head with medication
- Hold eyelids open (using palm of hand holding medication bottle)
- Apply one drop onto cornea or conjunctiva
- Apply ointment into fornix or onto the eye itself
- Avoid touching bottle/tube on animal fur (results in contamination)
- Gently occlude nasolacrimal punctae
- Prevent rubbing in immediate post-medication period
- Apply drops before ointments
- Leave 10 minutes between subsequent medications

See chapter 2 for further details and illustrations

Figures 2.1 (p. 15) and 4.8 show the application method. If the patient reacts differently from usual to the application of medication (for example, it suddenly wants to rub or vocalises), this should be noted on the hospital records and the clinician alerted.

If special topical agents are being used to treat a patient (e.g. home-formulated fortified antibiotic drops or autologous serum), extra care is needed with their handling. They should be refrigerated and replaced frequently (according to the clinician's instructions, but usually every 24–48 hours since they do not contain preservatives).

Systemic medication is given in the same way in all patients. However, care must be exercised with oral administration. Tablets in the food is the preferred method if the animal is eating well. However, if the tablets need to be administered directly, bear in mind that this might be painful for the patient. In a fully opened mouth, the vertical ramus of the mandible impinges on the retrobulbar tissues, which can be very painful in certain diseases (e.g. retrobulbar abscess or cellulitis and glaucoma). In these situations it is often better to give injections. Care must also be exercised if the patient has a deep corneal ulcer—struggling to avoid a tablet will increase blood pressure and intraocular pressure, which could result in the ulcer rupturing. If there is any concern that this could happen, the tablets should not be given and

the nurse should check with the ophthalmologist regarding an alternative route of medication.

If an intravenous catheter is placed it should be maintained as per general nursing guidelines.

Specific nursing instructions

There are some general considerations for ophthalmic patients which should be kept in mind. These include avoiding situations which could compromise the eye disease—mainly anything which could increase intraocular pressure. This is obviously important in patients with glaucoma, but is also of concern in patients with corneal ulcers, those which have undergone or are awaiting intraocular surgery and patients with uveitis. Situations which could increase intraocular pressure include coughing, barking (move the dog or place a blanket over the kennel door), pulling on the lead (use a chest harness or lead across the chest instead, Fig. 4.3) and taking the rectal temperature. Care should be exercised during jugular venepuncture—the positioning required together with occlusion of the jugular veins can increase intraocular pressure.

Some patients will require specific monitoring. For example, a dog with glaucoma might require its intraocular pressures to be taken every 2–3 hours, or a dog with keratoconjunctivitis sicca might require daily Schirmer tear test readings to be performed. Hypertensive cats might require blood

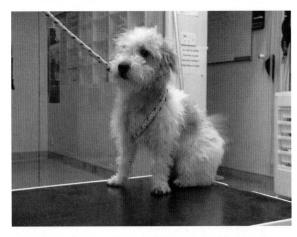

Fig. 4.3 Lead placed across chest to prevent animal pulling on the neck and resulting in an increase in intraocular pressure.

pressure measurement during their hospitalisation. The nurse can perform these tests (see Chapter 3). Other monitoring might include checking that the patient's eyes become moist on eating following a parotid duct transposition, or gentle massage of the face of such patients to encourage saliva flow up the parotid duct into the eye.

Nursing of diabetic patients will be encountered frequently in ophthalmic practice. In addition to their ocular medication, such patients will require specific feeding, insulin injections and monitoring of blood-glucose levels. Water intake should be measured, and they should be given frequent opportunities to urinate. Reference to general medical nursing texts will give further information.

Pain assessment

When giving medication and during general observation, it is important to establish whether the patient is in any discomfort from the eye(s). Sometimes this will be obvious: the eye will be closed with increased lacrimation and the patient will appear generally 'depressed' (i.e. quiet, inappetant, etc., Fig. 4.4). Hiding under covers, pressing the head against the kennel sides and attempts at rubbing also indicate pain or at least discomfort which should be addressed. Consider whether a human would be in any pain or discomfort with the same condition, and if they would be, it is usually safe to assume that the patient will be as well. Some

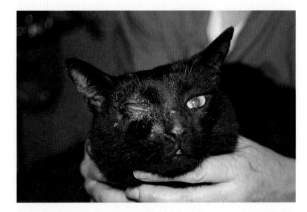

Fig. 4.4 Painful eye—the right eye of this cat is held closed, significant discharge is present together with some periorbital swelling.

patients will not appear to be in overt pain, but will demonstrate it on handling (e.g. shying away when approached from the affected side of the face or when the eye is gently cleaned). Any change in behaviour which could indicate pain should be reported to the clinician. If in any doubt regarding the degree of discomfort or pain, it is far better to provide analgesia and assess the response of the patient rather than leaving them in possible pain. A combination of opiates and NSAIDs are effective for most ocular pain and are discussed further in Chapter 6. Topical anaesthetics should be confined to diagnostic use; they damage corneal epithelium and should not be used for treating painful eyes.

Preventing self-trauma

The first thing to consider in preventing self-mutilation is why the animal wants to rub in the first case. Adequate pain relief will reduce the risk of self-trauma, as will keeping the patient comfortable (e.g. cleaning any discharge, ensuring a warm dry bed, etc.).

As briefly mentioned earlier, bedding can be ideal for the patient to rub against and care must be taken to avoid this. The choice of bedding is also important; for example, it should not shed fibres.

Some ophthalmologists dislike Elizabethan collars as they can unduly stress a patient. The patient can also bang the collars and jar their face and eyes, with the potential for damage. Such collars should never be used as an excuse for insufficient monitoring. Those used for ophthalmic patients preferably should be clear plastic rather than totally opaque, and the cone should not extend beyond the nose. Shorter collars still prevent the animal from reaching the eye(s) and causing damage (Fig. 4.5). An alternative method of preventing self-mutilation is the use of foot bandages. Well-padded dressings on the front feet (and occasionally the back ones as well) will prevent damage should the animal try to rub the eye(s) (Fig. 4.6). General nursing care for these will include keeping them dry, checking for discomfort and changing them as necessary. Cats do not tolerate these bandages well and so require Elizabethan collars more frequently. Collars should be

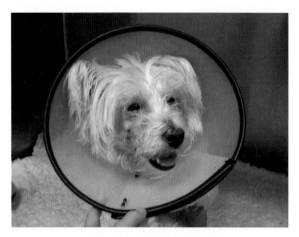

Fig. 4.5 Elizabethan collar to prevent self-trauma.

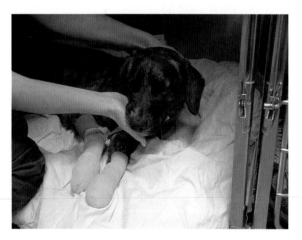

Fig. 4.6 Foot bandages to prevent damage to the eyes.

removed while the patient is eating since many cats will not feed if wearing them.

Patients are most likely to self-traumatise in the few minutes following topical medication or cleansing of the eyes. Thus, they should be closely monitored during this period. Some form of distraction (e.g. feeding, taking a walk or grooming) can be employed to prevent rubbing.

Infectious diseases

Some ophthalmic patients might be suffering from infectious disease, and as such it is important to consider barrier nursing. Cats present more frequently than dogs with infectious ocular disease—

the cat flu complex with feline herpes virus, *Chlamydophila* and possible Calici virus all spring to mind. In addition, feline immunodeficiency virus, feline leukaemia virus and feline panleukopaenia virus can be present in patients with ocular disease. Infectious diseases presenting with ocular signs in dogs include distemper and more exotic diseases such as leishmaniasis and erlichiosis, which are becoming increasingly prevalent in the UK as more and more animals are travelling abroad. The methods of nursing these patients (barrier nursing) will be similar. In addition, attention must be drawn to the method of transmission of infections—for example, via discharges (including ocular discharge) or by indirect contact with fomites. If the latter, any objects with which the patient has had contact (the cage, bowls, bedding, etc.) must be thoroughly disinfected before being used by another patient or, discarded. Disposable products should be used wherever possible. See Chapter 7 for more information on the specific infectious diseases encountered in ophthalmic practice.

DISCHARGE FROM THE HOSPITAL

When the patient is ready for discharge from the hospital, it is important that the owners fully understand what is expected of them in the way of aftercare. The clinician will have explained the nature of the animal's problem and discussed any diagnostic or surgical procedures which have been undertaken. Animals are often discharged with one or more medicines, and it is the nurse's responsibility to ensure that the owners are competent at giving these. Discharge instructions should be discussed prior to the release of the patient—as soon as owners see their pet they usually forget any further information given! When the owners come to collect their pet they should be taken into a consulting room and aftercare discussed. Written instructions are preferable (Fig. 4.7). If the animal has undergone surgery and is discharged the same day, monitoring for what to expect after general anaesthesia should be discussed.

Specific ophthalmic aftercare will consist of gently cleansing the eye and the application of

Post-operative eye care

Aftercare Sheet for ....……………......DATE..................

Your pet has just undergone surgery for an eye condition. These instructions are designed as a guide for caring for your pet in the post-operative period - it is important that you follow them closely since attention to detail can make all the difference to success or failure of the operation undertaken.

Make sure that a warm bed is provided away from any disturbance by people or other pets. It is important that your pet is kept relatively quiet for several days or even weeks following surgery. This means that dogs should have lead exercise only and cats should be kept indoors with a litter tray provided. You will be given specific advice for your animal, but stick to these instructions until informed otherwise.

OPERATION SITE - handle the eye(s) as little as possible. Gently clean away any discharge with damp cotton wool and apply treatment if dispensed. If the area is causing irritation, looks sore or is discharging excessively please seek veterinary advice immediately. If you have been supplied with an Elizabethan collar use it! Some patients have foot bandages instead to prevent self-trauma from rubbing - the nurse will give you instructions about keeping these dry and how often they need to be changed.

STITCHES - most sutures in and around the eye are soluble so do not need removing - however on occasions they do need taking out after 10 - 14 days.

MEDICATION   Dispensed ☐   Not dispensed ☐

OINTMENT / DROPS - apply to LEFT / RIGHT / BOTH eyes as follows

...................................to be applied............... times daily for................ days/until re-exam
...................................to be applied............... times daily for................ days/until re-exam
...................................to be applied............... times daily for................ days/until re-exam
....
Always leave at least 5 – 10 minutes between different drops and apply drops before ointment if you have both

TABLETS
.... to be given .... times daily for............... days
.... to be given .... times daily for............... days

COMMMENTS...
....
....
....
RE-EXAMINATION..

Fig. 4.7 Discharge instruction sheet.

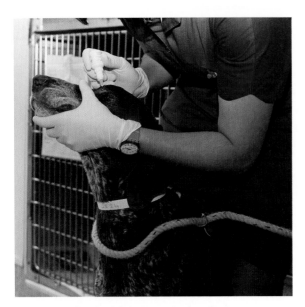

Fig. 4.8 Application of ointment wearing gloves.

drops and/or ointments. The nurse should make sure that the owner knows how to do this, and how frequently. Get the owner to demonstrate applying the medication to ensure proficiency. Ensure that the owner will be able to medicate as requested—every 8 hours for three-times-daily medication, every 6 hours for four-times-daily and so on. Check that there will be sufficient medication to last until the next check-up is due (this will help with owner compliance). If there are any special instructions for the medication (e.g. keeping it in the fridge or using gloves to apply, Fig. 4.8), confirm that the owner understands and will comply. It is also important to ensure that the owner knows which eye to medicate: if the instructions refer to the right eye it is the patient's right eye and not the one on the right as the owner faces the pet. It is very common for owners to get this simple fact confused! If the animal has foot bandages or an Elizabethan collar to prevent self-trauma, the care of these (e.g. removal of collar for feeding) should be considered.

The nurse should also let the owner know what to expect over the coming days—for example, when the animal will regain vision following cataract surgery, or when the swelling can be expected to reduce following cryosurgery for distichiasis. The owner should also be informed of when to contact the veterinary surgeon if they have any concerns,

and the date for a re-check appointment. Only when all of this has been discussed should the animal be brought to the owner.

LOOKING AFTER A BLIND PET

Unfortunately, some ocular conditions result in untreatable blindness. Examples include generalised progressive retinal atrophy, sudden acquired retinal degeneration, glaucoma and hypertension. Owners are often devastated to learn that their beloved pet will never see again. Sometimes their immediate reaction is to have their pet euthanased. Client education is an essential part of ophthalmic nursing. Owners may change their initial views regarding their blind pet if given a better understanding of the nature of the condition, and if helped to realise that blindness need not preclude a happy, fulfilled life. Reminding them that blind people still have a good life is useful! Dogs and cats rely on their senses of hearing and smell far more than humans, and so the loss of sight is usually less debilitating to them than it would be for us. Animals tend to sniff something unfamiliar, whether normally sighted or not; they recall how things smell rather than what things look like! Owners need to remember that it is far worse for them to watch their pet gradually adapt than it is for the pet to adjust. The pet does not wake up in the morning wondering how much worse its vision will be that day! And when they bump into a table one day they will quickly remember where it is and avoid it the next time.

How a pet reacts to becoming blind depends on many factors. These include the rapidity of the loss of vision, the age of pet, its temperament and its general training and ability to learn. If the blindness occurred gradually over several months, they adjust very well. Sometimes owners are not even aware that their pet is totally blind. Sudden onset conditions, such as retinal detachments, are more debilitating initially, and it takes a few weeks for the pet to adjust. Older pets will be familiar with their surroundings and probably less active than younger ones and, as such, adapt well. An exception to this is seen in very elderly patients in which there may be some cognitive function problems (senility). Nervous animals can take longer to adjust and are often initially unwilling to engage with the outside world, while bolder animals rarely have problems in this area. Well-trained dogs will respond quickly and learn new commands, and will have fewer problems with losing sight.

If the blind pet seems initially depressed (e.g. sleeping more, less interest in toys and games and unwilling to go for walks), the owner needs to gently encourage them to interact again. However, they should not be over protective. Training rather than smothering is important so that the pet retains a degree of independence. Some pets react better if there is another animal in the house, giving them some competition. Dogs which are sole pets might benefit from being walked with another friendly dog (so long as it is not too boisterous).

Animals will have a 'mental map' of their home environment: the house, garden and routine walks or territory. Owners should be instructed to alter this as little as possible. Furniture, the pet's bed, feeding and water bowls and litter tray for cats should not be moved. Children's toys should not be left lying around. Some people find that using scent marks (such as citronella or aromatherapy oils) on the door jams (at pet height) or on furniture will help to orientate the pet and allow it to avoid walking into the wrong side of the door, for example. Dogs in particular can find it difficult to go downstairs. They are usually happy to go up since they can feel for the next step, but on coming down do not know when they are getting to the bottom and often fall down the last few stairs. Having a mat at the bottom with a different texture to the stairs themselves can assist, since they soon learn to keep going down until they feel the different surface.

Hazards in the garden should be kept to a minimum. Low branches should be cut back, and roses or brambles should not be accessible. Ponds (and swimming pools) should be fenced off and any potentially dangerous walls or steep slopes made safe. The garden should be escape-proof.

Dogs should be allowed out for walks. Keeping to the same route each day will mean that they remain confident. They are creatures of habit anyway and this is emphasised more in blind dogs. A flexible lead is ideal to give them a degree of freedom while at the same time keeping some security and contact. If they are let off the lead it should be in a large, safe open space. It is useful to teach a 'danger' word to call out when the dog is rushing towards a tree or stream, for example, such that they quickly stop. They might also need teaching to go up and down kerbs and steps again. Some people find that having a bell, or jangling the house keys in their pocket, will reassure the pet that they are close by, such that the dog does not suddenly panic and feel abandoned.

Blind cats might still want to go outside and, providing they are familiar with the garden and local environment, this can be allowed. Some owners only let their blind cat out when they can supervise—just in case the cat gets frightened and runs off, or gets lost or injured. Cats might need to be guided to the cat flap (or litter tray if they do not go out).

Play should be continued with both dogs and cats. Toys with bells or squeakers, noisy clockwork mice or catnip toys are ideal. Balls should be rolled along rather than thrown so that the pet can hear the sound and follow accordingly. Food games (e.g. toys with treats hidden within) are also useful.

If the nurse spends some time discussing these points with owners, they are far more likely to accept the change in circumstance with their pet and continue to interact such that both pet and owner retain a good relationship and happy lives!

BIBLIOGRAPHY AND FURTHER READING

Bowden C, Masters J, eds. Textbook of veterinary medical nursing. Edinburgh: Butterworth Heinemann; 2003.
Lane DR, Cooper B, eds. Veterinary nursing. 3rd edn. Oxford: Butterworth Heinemann; 2003.

Moore AH, ed. BSAVA manual of advanced veterinary nursing. Gloucester: British Small Animal Veterinary Association; 1999.

5 Surgical nursing: equipment, instruments and the duties of the ophthalmic theatre nurse

INTRODUCTION

The general principles of ophthalmic surgery are to maintain optimum ocular comfort and eyelid function, to retain vision and to effect a cosmetic appearance. Unfortunately, many adnexal problems seen in our patients, especially in pedigree dogs, are related to their breed standard ('diamond eye' in the Saint Bernard, the excessive facial wrinkles in the Shar-pei, etc.). The owners' perception of what constitutes a cosmetic appearance can be at odds with the surgeon's opinion regarding ocular comfort and function. This is discussed further in the chapter on general ophthalmic conditions, but the role of the nurse in explaining and reassuring owners why certain procedures are necessary for their pet is very important. For example, owners can be concerned that the surgery will change the cosmetic appearance of their pet. Client education by the nurse will help allay these fears. For all ophthalmic surgery, we should remember that the tissues of the adnexa and eye itself are extremely delicate. Thus, the basic surgical principles of precise incisions, gentle tissue handling and accurate placement of sutures are paramount if a successful outcome is to be achieved. The use of inappropriate instruments or suture material can lead to unsatisfactory and disappointing results, and so the surgical nurse should be fully aware of the procedure to be undertaken and able to provide the surgeon with the appropriate equipment. A list of ophthalmic suppliers (including equipment, instruments and disposables) can be found in Appendix 3.

THE SURGICAL ENVIRONMENT

Strict attention to general hygiene is as important with ocular surgery as it is with any other surgical procedure. Some procedures are not strictly aseptic—for example, parotid duct transposition when both the oral cavity and the conjunctival sac are involved in the procedure, along with dissection of the duct itself. In this instance, the surgical

Table 5.1 Theatre preparation checklist

- Damp dusting—all surfaces and equipment should be wiped with a suitable disinfectant prior to the day's surgery
- Position operating table and place heat pads/positioning cushions etc. as required
- Check operating lights are functioning properly
- Check anaesthetic equipment
- Remove covers from operating microscope, check the bulbs are working and position
- Place surgical kits and disposables ready for opening and use
- Between patients—remove used instruments to preparation area for cleaning, wipe over all surfaces again (clean floor if necessary), reposition table and equipment, prepare instruments and disposables for the next procedure
- Once surgery finished for the day thoroughly clean theatre—wash floor and walls as well as all surfaces and equipment. Separate cleaning utensils should be available solely for theatre use

kit should contain sufficient instruments so that those entering the mouth can be discarded for the rest of the procedure to avoid contamination. The surgical nurse can liaise with the surgeon to make sure that the right instrument kits are available. Other types of ocular surgery require very strict asepsis. These include intraocular surgery, such as phacoemulsification for cataract extraction, intraocular lens placement and corneal transplantation. If bacterial contamination occurs with this type of surgery, the end result can be disastrous (i.e. loss of the eye). Therefore, both meticulous surgical preparation and an appropriate sterile theatre are required. Ideally, there should be a separate theatre dedicated for ophthalmic surgery, but unfortunately this is often not possible. Large equipment such as the operating microscope will remain in theatre, and if the room is used for other procedures, care must be taken to prevent it from being knocked (which could damage the internal optics). An outline of theatre preparation is provided in Table 5.1.

THEATRE EQUIPMENT

Good illumination and magnification are essential for ophthalmic surgery. For extraocular surgery, normal surgical lights are adequate (two should be positioned to avoid any shadows). Some procedures can be performed without magnification (e.g. entropion surgery), but spectacle or head-mounted magnifying loupes (Fig. 5.1) are helpful for procedures such as replacing prolapsed nictitans glands. Some magnifying loupes have an integrated head-mounted light source which projects the light exactly where the surgeon is looking.

For corneal and intraocular surgery, an operating microscope is required (Fig. 5.2). These vary tremendously in size and level of sophistication and, therefore, cost! All have integrated lighting, and many have spare bulbs included in the unit. If spares are not provided, one should always be available in case the bulb fails during a procedure. The most basic operating microscopes are table-mounted and provide limited functions, just one or two levels of magnification which must be altered manually. Floor or ceiling mounted models are more complex

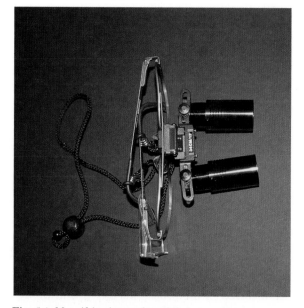

Fig. 5.1 Magnifying loupes for ophthalmic surgery.

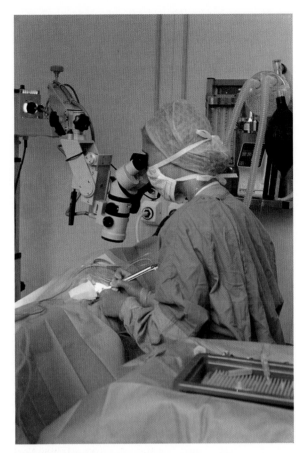

Fig. 5.2 Operating microscope.

and are recommended if a significant number of microsurgical procedures will be undertaken.

Many different companies supply microscopes, but all have similar features. A series of adjustable arms enables accurate positioning over the patient's eye. The distance between the patient and the head of the microscope is fixed by the optics of the machine. Focus is usually controlled via a foot switch, which can incorporate a zoom feature and side to side (X–Y) movement as well. Some older or less complex machines need to be moved manually, and plastic handles which can be sterilised are provided to enable the surgeon to reposition during the procedure. Many microscopes have a second viewing port for an assistant, which can be monocular or binocular. In addition, camera and video attachments are available for teaching purposes and for recording procedures. Magnification is usually in the range from 5–30×.

Since operating microscopes are so large, they remain in theatre at all times. A plastic cover is provided which should be washed as necessary. It is removed prior to use, and the microscope should be damp-dusted and switched on to check that it is functioning properly in advance of the day's surgery.

Since ophthalmic surgeons sit while operating, a good chair is essential. The chair should be of adjustable height (foot-operated hydraulic controls are ideal), with lockable casters to allow easy movement. Some chairs have a backrest which can be rotated for the surgeon to use as an arm rest during microsurgery. Other chairs incorporate a tilting seat to allow some lower back support while the surgeon leans forwards during surgery (Fig. 5.3).

Other items of equipment which might be required in theatre during ophthalmic surgery include phacoemulsification machines, lasers, cryosurgery equipment, electrolysis machines and electrocautery units. These are generally stored in the preparation room and brought into theatre only when required, unless too bulky to be moved easily.

Several types of phacoemulsification machine are available. The surgeon will chose the machine most suitable for practice needs, and specialised nurse training is required to learn how to set up and clean this expensive equipment. Further details of phacoemulsification can be found in Chapter 8.

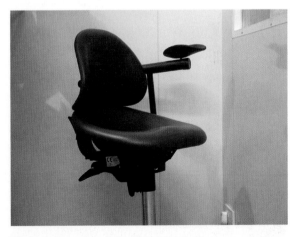

Fig. 5.3 Surgeon's chair with tilting back support and arm rest.

Table 5.2 Ophthalmic lasers and their indications

Type of laser	Indications
Diode	Glaucoma (cyclophotocoagulation) Retinal detachment surgery Limbal and uveal melanoma surgery Rupture of iris cysts Iridotomy
Nd-YAG*	Same indications as for diode
CO_2	Distichiasis removal Superficial keratectomy
Excimer	Superficial keratectomy (used in man for correction of myopia)

* Nd-YAG, neodymium:yttrium-aluminium-garnet

Lasers are becoming more common in ophthalmic practice. The different types available are listed in Table 5.2, together with some indications for their use. Due attention to health and safety issues must be paid whenever lasers are in operation.

Cryosurgery is used in veterinary ophthalmology for a variety of conditions. These include distichiasis, glaucoma, certain tumours (most commonly melanomas and squamous cell carcinomas) and the removal of subluxated and luxated lenses. Specific treatments are discussed further in Chapters 7 and 8. Both nitrous oxide and liquid nitrogen can be used, and a variety of probes and spray nozzles is available depending on the procedure undertaken (Fig. 5.4). Liquid nitrogen is colder than nitrous oxide, and shorter freezing times result. However, it is potentially more of a hazard, and extreme care should be taken if filling the hand-held thermos-type units.

Electrolysis (electroepilation) is used to treat distichiasis, ectopic cilia and trichiasis. Low levels of electric current are directed into the hair follicles to destroy them and prevent regrowth. The needle must be accurately placed directly into the hair follicle, and magnification is essential. Removal of the hair from the follicle with the electrolysis needle is usually an indication that the current has been placed successfully. Electrolysis can be time-consuming. Both battery powered and mains units are available. New needles must be used for each patient.

Electrocautery units are sometimes used for ocular surgery. Good haemostasis is essential—sometimes pressure alone is sufficient, but small battery powered portable units can be useful (Fig. 5.5). A variety of microtips is available for these, and the units can be sterilised and batteries inserted just before use. Alternatively, disposable sterile covers are also available. Standard wet-field electrocautery units (for coagulation not cutting) can be used, and some phacoemulsification machines have electrocautery facilities.

OPHTHALMIC SURGICAL INSTRUMENTS

Specific ophthalmic instruments are required for ocular surgery and these will be discussed below. It is not acceptable to employ general surgical instruments for ophthalmic use, apart from in gross procedures, such as enucleation. Standard surgical

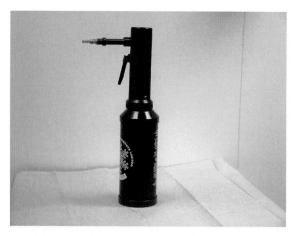

Fig. 5.4 Liquid nitrogen cryosurgery unit.

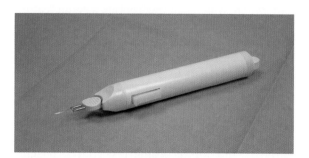

Fig. 5.5 Battery powered electrocautery unit.

kits for ophthalmic procedures would include a minimum of two types: extraocular (e.g. for eyelid and third eyelid surgery) and corneal/ intraocular kits. Separate kits for cataract surgery can be made up, or a small set of 'cataract instruments' can be packaged separately and opened in addition to the corneal/intraocular kit when required. A further kit containing larger instruments for enucleation can be packed (or a general surgery kit used instead). A supply of spare instruments packaged individually will also be required. Lists of suggested instruments to be included in pre-prepared packs are detailed in Tables 5.3, 5.4 and 5.5.

Instruments for ophthalmic surgery are designed to be manipulated with minimal movement by the surgeon: the upper arms and forearms remain still while the wrists and hands are used to manoeuvre the instruments. There are several differences in design from those for general surgery.

Table 5.3 Suggested instruments to be included in extraocular and corneal/intraocular instrument packs

Instrument	Use
Basic general ophthalmic kit (extraocular)	
Straight scissors	Cutting skin and canthotomy
Fine rat tooth forceps	Holding skin and conjunctiva
Steven's tenotomy scissors	Cutting conjunctiva
St Martins tying forceps	Holding conjunctiva and sutures
Needle holders (e.g. Castroviejo, without catch)	Suturing
Fine mosquito haemostats—curved and straight—3 pairs	Stabilising the globe and for haemostasis
Eyelid speculum	Provide globe exposure
Chalazion clamp	Stabilise lid margins
Blade handle (Bard–Parker)	Sharp incision
Towel clamps (2–4)	Stabilise drapes
For corneal and intraocular surgery	
Beaver handle	Corneal incision
Eyelid speculum	Globe exposure
Small straight scissors	Canthotomy
Tenotomy scissors (Steven's or Westcott's)	Conjunctival cutting
Corneal scissors (universal or right and left handed)	Enlarging corneal incision
Iris scissors	Cutting iris
Corneal micro forceps (Colibri)	Handling cornea
Tying forceps (St Martins)	Handling delicate suture material
Vectis	To remove luxated lenses
Delicate needle holders	To handle tiny needles
Mosquito forceps (straight and curved—3 pairs)	Stabilise the globe and provide haemostasis
Towel clamps/serrafines (4)	Secure drapes

Table 5.4 Extra instruments for cataract surgery

Instrument	Use
Keratome	Fixed length incision
Utrata capsule forceps	Capsulorhexis
Hydrodissection cannulae	Separating lens nucleus and cortex
Vannus scissors (straight or curved)	Cutting lens capsules
Nucleus rotator/phaco cleaver	Lens manipulation
Callipers	Measure incision for IOL* insertion
IOL introducer and forceps	Manipulation of IOL*

* IOL, intraocular lens

Table 5.5 Suggested instruments for an enucleation kit

- Allis tissue forceps
- Adson–Brown forceps
- Eyelid speculum
- Curved and straight haemostatic forceps
- Curved and straight mosquito haemostatic forceps
- Metzenbaum scissors
- Enucleation scissors
- Tenotomy scissors
- Bard parker scalpel handle
- Towel clamps
- Needle holders

the hand or wrist position does not need to be altered to reopen the instrument. A pin-stop may be present to prevent excessive pressure on closure, leading to damage to the delicate tips. Instruments which only operate in one direction (e.g. corneal scissors) often have flat handles, while those which require rotation during use (e.g. needle holders) may have rounded handles. General ophthalmic instruments are 120–140 mm in length, while microsurgical instruments are shorter, usually 100 mm (so that they do not touch the bottom of the microscope during the procedure). It is the surgical tips which need to be small, not the whole instrument, since it still needs to fit comfortably in the surgeon's hand!

They are light-weight—made either with materials such as titanium, or with holes in the handles to minimise weight (Fig. 5.6). They are also designed to be held in a pencil grip, with a similar diameter to that of a pen or pencil for ease of handling. Since the surgeon is often operating with the assistance of a surgical microscope, there is a need for tactile feedback. The surgeon often cannot see the instrument handles, just the tips. Ridges, knurling or flattening of the handles can be useful, and these variations also help to prevent slippage and can indicate the correct finger placement for holding and use. Instruments can have a slightly dulled or dark finish to reduce the scatter of reflected light under the microscope. In addition, ophthalmic instruments are often sprung so that

Eyelid specula

Eyelid specula (singular is speculum) are essential in veterinary ophthalmic surgery for a wide range of procedures. They are used to retract the lids and enhance exposure to the conjunctiva, cornea and globe. They should be strong enough to retract the lids easily but sufficiently lightweight to prevent direct pressure on the globe. They should not have large protruding ends around which sutures can become caught. Barraquer wire eyelid specula are common and come in paediatric and adult sizes. The former are useful for cats and small dogs. Larger breeds may require the Castroviejo-type of eyelid speculum, which has a screw to adjust the width of opening of the blades. Different lengths of blade are available depending on the eyelid length of the patient—smaller ones are required if a canthotomy is not performed. The blades are tucked under the lids in the closed position (or with the Barraquer speculum held closed) and gently opened to the required position. Figure 5.7 shows the two commonly used types of eyelid speculum.

Tissue forceps

Forceps are used for grasping eyelid skin, conjunctiva and corneal wound edges, and for the epilation of cilia. Different designs of instrument are available for each application. Microsurgical

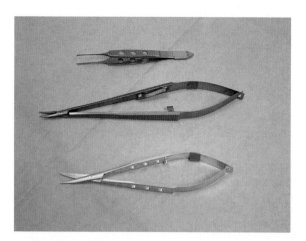

Fig. 5.6 Ways to lighten ophthalmic instruments with holes in handles and the use of titanium (needle holders in middle of photo) to reduce weight.

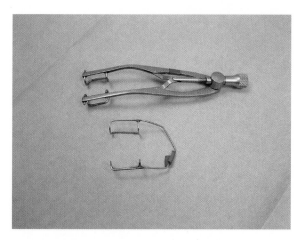

Fig. 5.7 Eyelid speculae—Castroviejo and Barraquer types.

forceps usually have angled tips (which help surgical visibility down the microscope). Forceps should be light enough to cause minimal damage to the tissue being grasped, while being strong enough such that they are not bent or damaged by the tissue. A tying platform can be incorporated close to the tip to allow suture material to be grasped without being damaged by the instrument tips themselves. It is essential that the instrument tips contact each other completely and in perfect alignment on digital closure. Forceps for conjunctival use usually have 1 × 2 teeth. However, these can cause button-hole tears in the delicate conjunctiva, and it may be preferable to use von Graefe forceps instead (Fig. 5.8) which have 10–14 fine

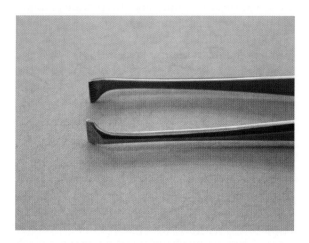

Fig. 5.8 Von Graefe's forceps—magnification showing the instrument tips.

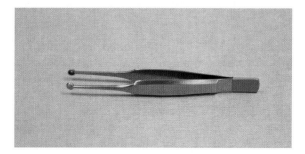

Fig. 5.9 Bennett's cilia forceps with rounded tips.

teeth allowing greater tension and holding ability but with reduced risk of tearing or conjunctival damage. However, these are too large for microsurgical procedures. Serrated tips on dressing forceps can be small enough for microsurgery and increase the surface area for grasping without the need to enlarge the instrument tips.

Cilia forceps have smooth blunt tips for grasping and removing aberrant lashes. Bennett's cilia forceps (Fig. 5.9) have rounded tips to prevent accidental damage to the lid margins, while Whitfield cilia forceps have flat oblique tips.

Forceps for grasping the cornea, sclera and limbus require teeth to hold the fibrous tissue. These can be perpendicular (dog-toothed) or splay-ended (tips ending outwards). The latter provide better grasping on smooth surfaces.

Iris forceps have serrated tips or very fine teeth. They have slender tips and shafts to allow intraocular manipulation.

Lens capsule and capsulorhexis forceps are used during cataract surgery. They are used to hold the anterior lens capsule or to allow controlled tearing of it. They have slender shafts, which are often angled to reduce obscuring of the surgeon's field of view down the operating microscope. Specialised instruments for manipulating intraocular lens implants are also available, as well as intraocular forceps for grasping foreign bodies within the globe.

Mosquito forceps (haemostatic forceps) are used for haemostasis and to stabilise parts of the globe (e.g. limbus or third eyelid). It is usual to have a selection of straight and curved ones available, along with larger haemostats for general use. Steeply curved ones are available for enucleation procedures—to make clamping the optic nerve and vessels easier.

Knives

The most frequently used knives in ophthalmic surgery are the standard Bard–Parker handle and blades (No.s 11 and 15), and the Beaver handle and blades (No.s 64, 65 and 67 plus specialist blades). The latter are used for conjunctival and corneal incisions. Keratomes are diamond-shaped blades and are mainly used for cataract surgery. They either fit to the Beaver handles or come as separate disposable instruments, and provide an incision of accurate width (e.g. 3.2 mm for the introduction of the phacoemulsification needle). The diamond knife is a reusable scalpel blade and handle for corneal, limbal and scleral incisions. Although very expensive, with proper care it can last for many years. Restricted depth knives are useful for corneal surgery (e.g. superficial keratectomy and the removal of corneal sequestra). These have a rounded blade with a raised button such that the blade can only be inserted a small distance into the cornea. Figure 5.10 shows examples of ophthalmic knives.

Scissors

A wide variety of ophthalmic scissors is available. They differ in their tips (sharp, rounded or curved) and handles (ringed or spring-handled). For eyelid and conjunctival dissection, Steven's tenotomy

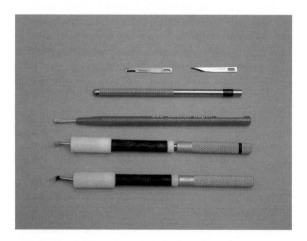

Fig. 5.10 Variety of surgical knives—Beaver blades and handle, fixed depth and standard keratomes.

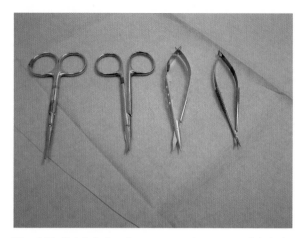

Fig. 5.11 Ophthalmic scissors—general purpose ophthalmic, Steven's tenotomy, Westcott's and microcorneal.

scissors are versatile, with either straight or slightly curved tips. A small pair of Metzenbaum scissors is useful for general eyelid skin dissection, while special enucleation scissors are available which have sharply curved blades and blunt tips. Corneal and corneoscleral scissors tend to have flat handles with springs rather than rings for holding them, allowing a greater control of cutting. Universal corneal scissors can cut in either direction, while left- and right-handed scissors allow the accurate enlargement of a corneal incision in both directions (and are available for both right- and left-handed surgeons). The length of handles and blades will be smaller for microsurgical scissors than for general ophthalmic ones. Iris scissors are small, delicate and very sharp with pointed, slightly angled tips. Tiny intraocular scissors, such as Vannus scissors, are used to cut the lens capsule during cataract surgery. Figure 5.11 shows some ophthalmic scissors.

Needle holders

Needle holders should be chosen according to the size of needle. They are often shaped similarly to corneal scissors, but with rounded, rather than flat, handles and a spring action such that they are open in the resting position. The tips can be straight or curved, with smooth or serrated surfaces. A locking mechanism can be present, which maintains the tips closed when a needle is grasped.

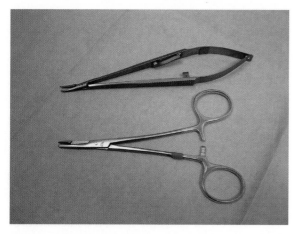

Fig. 5.12 Ophthalmic needle holders—Castroviejo and small Olsen–Hegar type.

These are suitable for larger sutures but not for microsurgical procedures, since the opening of the lock can jar the tips slightly affecting the precise positioning of the suture. Microsurgical needle holders without a lock usually possess a pin stop to prevent excessive compression of the handles damaging the tips. Needle holders are shown in Figure 5.12.

Miscellaneous instruments

Nettleships dilator

This is a small pencil-like instrument used to locate the nasolacrimal punctae prior to cannulation (Fig. 5.13). It is an invaluable instrument, both for diagnostic purposes in nasolacrimal flushing and during surgery for micro- or imperforate nasolacrimal punctae.

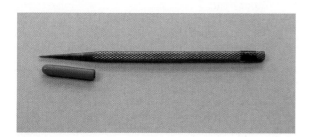

Fig. 5.13 Nettleship's dilator.

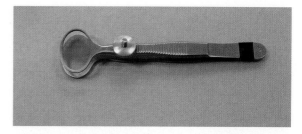

Fig. 5.14 Chalazion clamp.

Chalazion clamp

The Desmarre's chalazion clamp has two plates, one open and one solid, and a screw to tighten and fix the instrument on the lid (Fig. 5.14). It is useful in many procedures, including the excision of an eyelid mass, ectopic cilia removal and cryosurgery for distichia. It stabilises the lid, maintains haemostasis and protects the underlying globe from inadvertent damage. Various sizes are available.

Jaeger lid plate

This is a smooth plate used to stabilise the eyelid so that an incision can be made against the plate. This also protects the underlying globe.

Chalazion curette

Several sizes of Meyerhoefer chalazion curettes are available. They are small sharp curettes used to remove inspissated material from chalazia and are best employed in conjunction with a chalazion clamp.

Spatulae/retractors/hooks

Special instruments are available for various intraocular procedures and include spatulae, iris and extraocular muscle hooks, intraocular lens instruments and lens loops. Spatuale are used to manipulate the iris during intraocular surgery or to gently move the vitreous during cataract surgery. Iris repositors are similar. Various types are available with blunt or rounded blades. Iris hooks have angled, blunt ends, to gently retract the pupillary

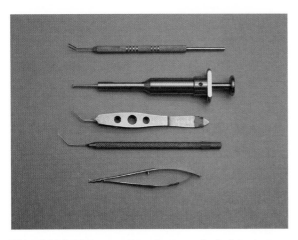

Fig. 5.15 Instruments sometimes used during cataract surgery—lens forceps, IOL introducer, Utrata forceps, nucleus rotator/phaco chopper, Vannus scissors.

margins of the iris. Muscle hooks are similar but much larger and can be placed beneath the extra-ocular muscles to allow globe rotation. Lens loops (e.g. Snellen vectis) are used during intracapsular lens extraction and occasionally for nuclear delivery during extracapsular extraction. They consist of a straight handle and open loop at the end to slide the lens from the anterior chamber. Various instruments are available to assist phacoemulsification—for example, the nucleus rotator, phaco chopper and capsule polisher. Nurses working in specialised ophthalmic practice will be familiar with the array of instruments required for intraocular surgery, some of which are shown in Figure 5.15.

Foreign body spud

A single- or double-ended instrument with sharp pointed tips is sometimes used to remove corneal or intraocular foreign bodies. However, many surgeons simply use two fine gauge hypodermic needles instead!

Callipers

During some intraocular procedures it is necessary to have exact measurements of tissues, and callipers are used for this. They are usually sterilised separately from the main ocular kits, or can

be included in the cataract kits since they are not used for every procedure.

Serrafine clamps

Small cross-action serrafine clamps are occasionally used to help stabilise the globe by attaching them to stay sutures.

INSTRUMENT STERILISATION

Sterilisation—the process of destroying all micro-organisms on an instrument—can be achieved by chemical (cold) or heat processes, and both can be used for most ophthalmic instruments. An autoclave using steam under pressure at a temperature of 121° C is routinely used. Ethylene oxide is also efficient and prevents the blunting of delicate surgical blades (such as corneal scissors) which occurs with repeated steam autoclaving. Appropriate attention to health and safety matters is essential if ethylene oxide is used.

Since ophthalmic instruments are so delicate, they should be packed in specially designed boxes which keep them separate from each other and secure. Both metal and plastic types are available. Those with silicone rubber 'fingers' to separate the instruments are ideal (Fig. 5.16). Individual instruments should have rubber tips placed on any sharp or delicate parts. It is usual to include a chemical indicator strip within the box, as well as in the outer wrapping, to ensure adequate sterili-

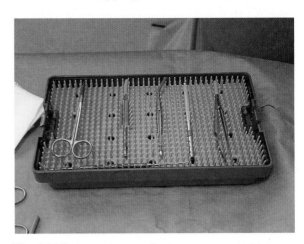

Fig. 5.16 Instrument storage box.

sation. Indicator tape is not a reliable method for checking sterilisation (it does not show that the correct time/pressure/temperature has been reached, only that exposure has occurred). Instrument boxes are wrapped in a paper or linen drape, placed in a self-seal sterilisation bag and labelled prior to sterilisation. They should be stored in a dedicated ophthalmic cupboard.

CARE OF OPHTHALMIC INSTRUMENTS

Since the instruments used for eye surgery are so delicate, it is important that special attention is taken with their handling and general care. They should not be jumbled in a used drape and left until later to be cleaned! Immediately upon cessation of surgery, the instruments should be gently placed in warm water with a mild non-corrosive instrument-cleaning agent. They should be placed such that no overlapping occurs, and hinged instruments should be opened. Each instrument should be gently scrubbed with a small soft brush (Fig. 5.17) and then rinsed with water (ideally distilled or deionised). They can be air-dried (spread out on a towel) or gently hand-dried with a lint-free cloth. Ultrasonic cleaning is efficient, but ophthalmic instruments rarely become so contaminated that regular ultrasonic cleaning is needed. If ultrasonic cleaning machines are employed, again it is mandatory that instruments are placed in the cleaning basket in a single, non-touching layer. Special instrument lubricants should be used if required after cleaning. The instruments should be checked to make sure they are working properly prior to

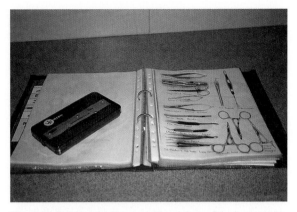

Fig. 5.18 Folder with lists and illustrations of the instruments found in each ophthalmic kit.

packing. Check that the tips of forceps meet properly and that hinges function smoothly. The surgeon should be made aware of any problems immediately. If a spare instrument is not available, the kit must be labelled to indicate that the instrument is missing. Damaged instruments can often be repaired by the manufacturer (or a certified repairer) for a fraction of the cost of replacements.

Surgical instruments can be identified with coloured plastic autoclavable tape to help identify the surgical pack to which they belong. Any such tape should be positioned such that it does not interfere with the functioning of the instrument. In addition, a list of the instruments for each kit should be provided. It is sometimes helpful to illustrate the instrument as well (placing them directly onto the glass top of a photocopier works well), and the copies can be included with the list (Fig. 5.18).

SUTURE MATERIAL

The choice of suture material for ophthalmic procedures will depend upon the type of tissue to be sutured (e.g. eyelid or cornea), the risk of contamination and the length of time for which support will be required. Surgeon preference will also be a factor. Needles and suture material should be of small gauge and, as such, sutures need to be placed close together. For this reason, absorbable sutures will sometimes be used in the skin (e.g. following entropion correction) since this removes the necessity to take out the sutures, which could

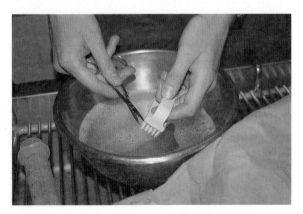

Fig. 5.17 Cleaning ophthalmic instruments.

Table 5.6 Suture material for ophthalmic surgery

Suture Type	Size	Use
Non absorbable		
Nylon (monofilament)	3-0–4-0	Stay sutures
		Occasionally skin
	8-0–10-0	Cornea
Silk (braided)	4-0–7-0	Eyelid skin
		Conjunctiva
Absorbable		
Polygalactin 910 (Vicryl, Ethicon)	4-0–6-0	Subcutaneous tissue
		Skin
	8-0–9-0	Conjunctiva
		Cornea
Polyglycolic acid (Dexon, Davis & Geck)	2-0–4-0	Subcutaneous tissue
		Subconjunctival tissue
Polydioxanone (PDS, Ethicon)	2-0–5-0	Subcutaneous tissue
		Subconjunctival tissue

Table 5.7 Needle design for ophthalmic surgery

Cross section tip shape		Features	Use
Cutting	△	Sharp point and sides Triangle in cross section Traumatic to tissue Difficult to accurately control depth	Skin
Reverse cutting	▽	Sharp point and sides Upside-down triangle in cross section Traumatic to tissue Difficult to accurately control depth	Skin
Taper point	⊘	Sharp point but smooth sides Little tissue trauma Not sharp enough for skin	Conjunctiva
Spatula tipped	⬭	Designed for use in lamellar tissue as remain in same plane and thus accurate placement is possible	Cornea

require sedation or even general anaesthesia. Soft sutures are required close to the eyes; corneal abrasion by sharp suture ends must be avoided. The choice of needle is also important. It is usual for these to be swaged-on to the suture. Taper-point needles are ideal for the conjunctiva but are not sharp enough for the skin, where reverse cutting needles are usually chosen. For corneal suturing, spatula-tip needles are employed, since these remain in the plane in which they are placed and can be accurately controlled by the surgeon.

Tables 5.6 and 5.7 show the suture materials and needles commonly used for ophthalmic surgery.

DISPOSABLE ITEMS FOR OPHTHALMIC SURGERY

These are listed in Table 5.8.

Table 5.8 Disposable items for routine ocular surgery

Disposable item	Use
Standard surgical blades (e.g. No. 15)	Eyelid and conjunctival incision
Beaver blades (Nos 64, 65 & 67)	Corneal incision
Restriction depth knives	Superficial keratectomy
Nasolacrimal cannulae—various sizes	Cannulating nasolacrimal punctae
2mL syringe	Flushing the cornea or nasolacrimal duct
BSS, Hartmann's or Ringer's solution	Intraocular irrigation
Celluose Spears	Microsurgical swabs
Soft gauze swabs (Topper, Johnson & Johnson)	Gently removing discharges
Suture material of appropriate size	Suturing cornea, conjunctiva or eyelids
Drapes—sticky plastic centre useful for corneal/intraocular surgery	Assist with aseptic surgical site
Microcautery	Haemostasis

Drapes

Normal draping material can be used for ophthalmic surgery. Both linen and disposable drapes can be employed. Fenestrated fabric drapes can be used, but since these are not water-resistant they are often reserved for extraocular procedures. Prepacked sterile disposable drapes are water resistant, and as such are employed for corneal and intraocular surgery where irrigating fluids are used. Many surgeons prefer drapes with a sticky plastic window which adheres to the skin around the eye. The surgeon then cuts into the plastic to expose the cornea. The drape can be folded back under the eyelids to prevent any stray hairs from entering the surgical site, and this provides a more aseptic surgical field than fabric or paper drapes

alone. Specialised drapes for cataract surgery include a pouch in the drape or a separate bag to collect excess irrigating fluid.

Swabs

It is essential that swabs used for ocular surgery are soft and lint-free (e.g. Topper swabs, Johnson & Johnson). Any fibres left in the ocular area could be irritating. For microsurgery, cellulose spears are advised. These come in packs of 5, 10 or 20 and are safe to dab the cornea, and can absorb intraocular fluids as necessary (Fig. 5.19).

Surgical blades

These were discussed on page 70 (under 'Knives').

Cannulae

Disposable plastic nasolacrimal cannulae should always be available. In addition, fine metal cannulae are used to irrigate the anterior chamber—a variety of both reusable and disposable types can be obtained. Specialised hydrodissection cannulae are used during cataract surgery.

Irrigating fluids

Sterile saline, Hartmann's solution and balanced salt solution (BSS) can all be used as irrigating

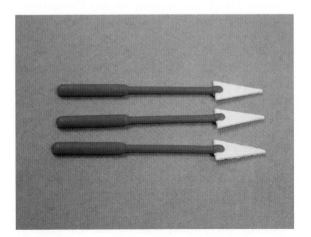

Fig. 5.19 Cellulose spears for specialised ophthalmic surgery.

fluids. Saline is usually restricted to cleansing procedures prior to surgery but can be employed to flush the cornea and conjunctival sac, or for checking nasolacrimal duct patency. It is not advised for intraocular surgery. Here it is more appropriate to use a solution which is similar in consistency to aqueous humour (i.e. Hartmann's, Ringer's or BSS). In addition to being balanced with regard to sodium and chloride content, these agents contain buffers such as bicarbonate which make them physiologically more similar to aqueous humour than saline alone. As such, they are non-irritating and cause minimal damage to delicate intraocular tissues such as the corneal endothelium.

MISCELLANEOUS ITEMS FOR OPHTHALMIC SURGERY

In addition to surgical instruments and disposable items, some other items need mentioning. These include positioning devices, contact lenses, collagen shields, tissue adhesives and specialised items for cataract and glaucoma surgery. The latter are discussed in Chapter 8. Here we will briefly mention those items needed for more routine procedures.

The positioning of the patient for ocular surgery is very important; the difference of only a few millimetres can affect the ease of access for the surgeon, especially during microsurgery. Most ophthalmologists prefer to use vacuum cushions to assist positioning. Small- and large-sized are available, but the smaller size is usually sufficient. Most general surgical suppliers can provide them. The patient's head is placed on the pillow and held in the desired position while the hand pump removes the air. The pillow is sealed and the pump removed. Occasionally sand bags are required as well, especially for dogs with long noses or heavy heads. These should be cleaned between patients (and separate from those used for radiography, for example).

Contact lenses (bandage soft contact lenses) are frequently used in dogs and cats, as well as horses. They provide ocular comfort during the healing of a corneal ulcer while protecting the delicate epithelium from being rubbed by the eyelids during blinking. Several sizes are available, and the width of the cornea and its angle of curvature should be carefully measured. Most suppliers provide an easy to use measuring card for this pur-

pose. In addition to treating corneal ulcers, contact lenses can be used for spastic entropion to relieve the blepharospasm, thus allowing the eyelid to return to its normal position.

Collagen shields can be used as a bandage during the healing of a corneal ulcer. They are supplied in individual sterile packets and need to be rehydrated fully before inserting into the eye. They dissolve in a few days.

Tissue adhesives can be used to treat corneal ulcers and are discussed in Chapter 2.

PREPARATION FOR SURGICAL PROCEDURES

The theatre nurse has an important role in the smooth running of the surgical list. In addition to liaising with surgeons, anaesthetists, kennel nurses and any other members of the team, the theatre nurse should ensure that theatre is ready for each procedure and that the appropriate instrument kits and any extra items which might be required are sterilised and ready for use.

Sorting the order of work

Following general surgical principles it is advisable to start with clean procedures, followed by clean-contaminated and then contaminated or 'dirty' operations. Thus, cataract surgery and other intraocular procedures would always be performed first. Corneal surgery might be next, followed by eyelid and nictitans surgery. Parotid duct transposition involves dissection into the mouth and thus would be performed later. Dirty procedures, such as retrobulbar abscess investigation, should be left until the end of the surgical list (or performed outside theatre). If a surgical emergency, such as a lens luxation, needs to be performed after less-clean operations, theatre should be thoroughly cleaned (and allowed to dry) before proceeding with the emergency.

Surgical preparation of the patient

Normally the patient will be starved prior to surgery (unless an emergency procedure) and

Table 5.9 Surgical preparation

Step	Agent used	Method
1	Fine clippers	Apply K-Y Jelly (Johnson & Johnson) to clipper blades so hairs stick to them
2	1:50 dilution povidine iodine solution	Use 5–10 ml syringe to flush conjunctival sac
3	Sterile saline, e.g. Aquaspray (Animalcare)	Use 5–10 ml syringe to flush conjunctival sac again
4	1:10 povidine iodine solution	On gauze free swabs (e.g. Topper, (Johnson & Johnson) to surgically prepare skin

should have been given the opportunity to empty bladder and bowels prior to premedication and induction of anaesthesia.

Clipping

Once anaesthetised, the patient can be prepared for surgery (Table 5.9). This should be done outside theatre in the preparation room. If the procedure is unilateral, the fellow eye should be protected with a lubricating gel or ointment (e.g. Lacrilube [liquid paraffin, Allergan] or Viscotears [Carbomer 980, Ciba Vision]). This is also applied to the surgical eye to protect it from damage by careless clipping and to reduce hair deposition in the conjunctival sac. Eyelashes should be cut with small sharp scissors. Applying some ophthalmic lubricant or KY Jelly (Johnson & Johnson) to the scissor blades prior to use will encourage the lashes to adhere to the scissors. Some surgeons do not clip further for corneal or intraocular surgery since any clipper rash which could develop might cause the animal to rub the eye. If the area is not clipped it is essential to use sticky drapes for the surgical procedure, tucking them under the eyelids to provide a sterile operating field. Obviously, clipping is essential for lid surgery. Water-based ointment (such as KY Jelly) can be applied to the fur which is to be removed so that it sticks to the clipper blades—these will need more frequent cleaning as a result but the production of stray hairs is markedly reduced. Sharp fine clipper blades (no bigger than No. 40) are required, and a separate blade dedicated to ophthalmic use is advised. The area clipped should be 2 cm beyond the expected surgical site. The lateral canthus should be clipped for any procedures which might require a canthotomy. Remember to be neat with the area clipped—the owners will notice this before they comment on any surgery! The skin around the eyes is usually quite loose and can be difficult to clip without snagging unless it is pulled tight during the procedure.

Preparation of the surgical site

After clipping the stray hairs should be removed. Light suction with a hand-held vacuum cleaner can be used but care must be taken not to damage the eye. Non-sterile gloves should be worn during surgical preparation to prevent contamination from the nurse's hands. Sterile saline on lint-free swabs (e.g. Topper Swabs [Johnson & Johnson], various sizes available) can be used to gently wipe the area, removing any remaining hairs.

The conjunctival sac is an external body surface with a normal population of flora, mainly Gram-positive bacteria but also viruses and fungi. This fact, along with the need for gentle handling during patient preparation to prevent swelling, bruising, corneal damage or chemical injury, is considered when choosing appropriate ocular disinfectants. Solutions of povidine–iodine (Pevidine solution, various manufacturers) are chosen to disinfect the surgical site. Dilutions are made in sterile saline or distilled water. Detergent-containing scrub solutions must not be used as they will damage corneal surfaces. Chlorhexidine solutions are also avoided as they are more irritant and can also damage the cornea and conjunctiva. Solutions containing alcohol must never be used near the eyes. A solution of 1:50 dilution of povidine–

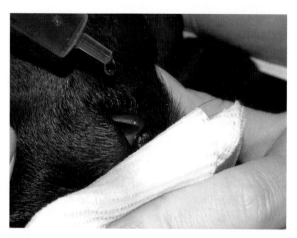

Fig. 5.20 Surgical preparation using diluted povidine–iodine solution.

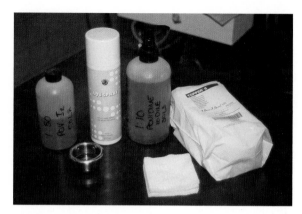

Fig. 5.21 Disinfectants used for ocular surgical preparation.

iodine solution is used to flush the conjunctival sac: a 5–10 ml syringe is used and refilled as required. If a suspected corneal rupture is present, povodine–iodine should not be used as it can be irritating to intraocular structures. The low 1:50 concentration retains virucidal, bactericidal and fungicidal activity with minimal damage to the ocular surfaces. The conjunctival fornix should be carefully flushed (Fig. 5.20). Sterile cotton buds or cellulose spears can be soaked in the 1:50 dilution and used to remove any mucous or debris from the conjunctival sac. Any residual ophthalmic ointments must be thoroughly removed as well. The antiseptic is then carefully flushed out with sterile saline solution or Hartmann's solution. At least 10 ml is used to flush the conjunctiva. The local skin is then cleansed with a 1:10 dilution of povidine-iodine solution on lint-free swabs. Care is taken to ensure that this does not come into contact with the cornea or conjunctiva.

If a bilateral procedure is being performed, the patient can be turned, with the newly cleansed eye protected by a clean dry lint-free swab while the second eye is similarly prepared. When the surgeon is ready to operate on the second eye the final skin preparation with the 1:10 dilution of povidine–iodine solution is repeated in theatre. It is not usually necessary to repeat the entire surgical preparation procedure unless known contamination has occurred. It is recommended to have dilutions of the preparation agents made up in bottles for ease of use. These should be replaced frequently (every 2–4 weeks) and are shown in Figure 5.21.

Positioning the patient

Once in theatre, the positioning of the patient can make an enormous difference to the ease of surgery. Thus, many ophthalmic surgeons will position the patient themselves prior to scrubbing-up. In general, the aim should be to have the cornea in the horizontal plane. This is achieved with the aid of vacuum cushions and washable sand-bags to elevate the nose while the patient rests in lateral recumbency. Dorsal recumbency is sometimes used for bilateral procedures, since the head can be repositioned without needing to move the whole animal. The suction-port for the vacuum bag should always be positioned so that the nurse can easily access it during the procedure if necessary. Care should be taken to protect the downside non-surgical eye (especially in brachycephalic patients). The forelegs should be pulled back away from the head so that they do not get in the way of the surgeon. If necessary, they can be secured with ties.

Theatre clothing

Obviously, all members of the theatre team will wear scrub suits, hats, masks and appropriate footwear. Surgical gowns for ophthalmic use can be reusable or disposable. If the former are used, the type with a nylon front panel which is water resistant is preferred; these prevent moisture strike-through and the associated risk of contamination. It is particularly important to consider this during intraocular surgery where large volumes of fluid are used for intraocular irrigation. Disposable non-woven gowns might be preferable for this type of procedure.

Gloves

Sterile gloves are mandatory for all ocular surgery. Powder-free gloves must be used, as the starch present in some gloves will act as a foreign body and cause a catastrophic inflammatory reaction in or around the eye. Special microsurgical gloves are available which have textured finger-tips, allowing better grip of the instruments.

Setting out instruments

Sometimes the surgeon will set out the instruments themselves, but a scrubbed nurse can do this. A sterile drape is placed over the clean trolley before the surgery kit is opened and placed on the trolley. The instruments which are likely to be used are laid out from left to right in their anticipated order of use—for example, scissors to cut the drape, eyelid speculum, instruments to place stay sutures, knife and so on. Instruments which might not be required should be safely left in the box. Sterile disposables, such as swabs, cannulae and sutures, can be opened. If the surgery is not going to start immediately, the trolley should be covered with a sterile drape until ready for use.

ROLE OF THE THEATRE NURSE

During surgery

Once the patient is prepped and positioned, the surgeon will scrub-up, gown and glove for surgery. The nurse will assist with this. If the instruments are not already laid out, the nurse will open the instrument kits and disposables for the surgeon. During the procedure the nurse can attend to non-sterile equipment, such as controls on the phacoemulsification or electrocautery machine, and fetch any extra items which might be required, such as fluids or further swabs.

Once the procedure has finished

Once the operation has been completed and the anaesthetist starts to recover the patient, the theatre nurse can clear away the instruments ready for cleaning and re-sterilisation. If the patient is due any topical medication immediately after surgery, this can be applied. The surgical site can be gently cleaned with sterile saline on soft, lint-free swabs. Any foot bandages to be used to reduce postoperative self-trauma can be applied now. However, Elizabethan collars should not be fitted until the patient is more fully recovered from anaesthesia. The theatre nurse should also check post-surgical instructions. If the patient is going home the same day, a discharge sheet should be completed. Alternatively, the hospital record sheet should be updated and any changes in medication noted together with special care instructions.

BIBLIOGRAPHY AND FURTHER READING

Gelatt KN, Gelatt JP. Handbook of small animal ophthalmic surgery. Volumes 1 and 2. Oxford: Pergamon; 1994.

Gelatt KN. Veterinary ophthalmology. 3rd edn. Philadelphia: Lippincott Williams & Wilkins; 1999.

Lane DR, Cooper B, eds. Veterinary nursing. 3rd edn. Oxford: Butterworth Heinemann; 2003.

Moore AH, ed. BSAVA manual of advanced veterinary nursing. Gloucester: British Small Animal Veterinary Association; 1999.

Moore M, ed. BSAVA Manual of veterinary nursing. Gloucester: British Small Animal Veterinary Association; 1999.

Petersen-Jones S, Crispin S, eds. BSAVA manual of small animal ophthalmology. 2nd edn. Gloucester: British Small Animal Veterinary Association; 2002.

6 Anaesthesia for ophthalmic surgery

CHAPTER SUMMARY

- Introduction
- Principles of anaesthesia
- Physiology and anaesthesia (pertaining to the eye)
- Preoperative assessment
- Anaesthetic plan
- Anaesthetic drugs
  Premedication
  Analgesia
  Induction
  Maintenance
  Muscle relexant anaesthesia
  Monitoring
  Recovery
- Anaesthesia in patients with diabetes mellitus
- Sedation for minor ophthalmic procedures
- Rabbit anaesthesia
- Equine anaesthesia

INTRODUCTION

The animal undergoing anaesthesia will always be under the direct care of the veterinary surgeon, and the nurse should always keep the surgeon informed of the condition of the animal throughout the procedure. Nurses must only undertake procedures which they feel competent to perform (under the supervision of the veterinary surgeon).

Qualified nurses should be competent to administer medication (including intravenous drugs and fluid therapy), prepare animals for anaesthesia and assist with its administration and with recovery. The veterinary surgeon remains responsible for the induction and maintenance, together with full recovery of the patients under their care. Thus, it is the surgeon's responsibility to assess whether the animal is fit for anaesthesia, and if so which agents should be used and at what doses. The veterinary surgeon should normally administer any controlled drugs such as methadone or morphine. However, the veterinary nurse can administer the pre-chosen premedication, administer anaesthetic agents (providing they are not incremental or 'to effect' but at a pre-calculated dose rate), keep an anaesthetic record, monitor clinical signs and maintain anaesthesia under the direct supervision of the veterinary surgeon. The role of the veterinary nurse during anaesthesia is outlined in Table 6.1. Although many of the techniques used are applicable to many anaesthetics, there are some specific differences which relate to ophthalmic surgery, and these will be discussed in this chapter.

PRINCIPLES OF ANAESTHESIA

The main reason for anaesthesia is to permit medical or surgical procedures to be undertaken. This

Table 6.1
The role of the veterinary nurse during the stages of anaesthesia
<ul><li>To ensure that the patient is prepared for anaesthesia according to the veterinary surgeon's instructions, e.g. appropriate eye drops have been given, intravenous catheter placed</li><li>To prepare an anaesthetic record sheet for the animal</li><li>To administer pre-anaesthetic medication as instructed by the veterinary surgeon</li><li>To observe the animal following administration of the premed</li><li>To prepare and check all necessary equipment for the anaesthetic</li><li>To assist the veterinary surgeon at all times</li><li>To monitor the patient during anaesthesia</li><li>To record all monitored parameters on the anaesthetic record sheet</li><li>To observe the patient during recovery</li><li>To administer any treatments requested by the veterinary surgeon</li></ul>

is highlighted in the Protection of Animals (Anaesthetics) Acts of 1954 and 1964, which state that 'carrying out of any operation with or without the use of instruments, involving interference with the sensitive tissues or bone structure of an animal, shall constitute an offence unless an anaesthetic is used in such a way as to prevent any pain to the animal during the operation'. Therefore, the control of pain is also a purpose of the anaesthetic. In addition, it can be used to facilitate examination by immobilising the animal (anaesthesia or sedation are used in fractious patients to reduce the risk of injury to both themselves and the staff involved) or if an animal is in significant pain, making clinical examination unethical (e.g. in an animal with a severe corneal injury). Anaesthetic agents are also used to control status epilepticus and for euthanasia, but these applications are rarely necessary as part of ophthalmic nursing.

Anaesthesia is generally classified as either local or general.

- **Local anaesthesia** relates to the elimination of sensation from a part of the body—the eye in our case. The local sensory (and/or motor) neurones of the peripheral nervous system are depressed with local anaesthesia. For the eye, we can use topical agents to numb the ocular surface, or regional nerve blocks (e.g. retrobulbar).

- **General anaesthesia** is the elimination of sensation by controlled, reversible depression of the central nervous system. External noxious stimuli result in reduced sensitivity and motor responses in anaesthetised animals. The perfect anaesthetic drug would induce reversible unconsciousness, analgesia and muscle relaxation without the depression of circulation and respiration. It would not be toxic to the patient and would not require metabolism prior to elimination. Unfortunately, such a single drug does not exist. However, by using 'balanced anaesthesia' we can aim to achieve these goals. Balanced anaesthesia involves the use of more than one drug to optimise the desired effects of anaesthesia, such as good muscle relaxation and rapid elimination from the body, while minimising the undesired effects such as respiratory and cardiac depression. Generally, a combination of injectable and inhalation agents is used to achieve the balance between unconsciousness (narcosis), analgesia and muscle relaxation.

The anaesthetic period is divided into five stages. These are outlined below and are discussed in greater detail later in the chapter.

1. Preoperative period

The veterinary surgeon examines the animal and decides on the appropriate anaesthetic protocol. This will be based upon the health of the animal, procedure to be undertaken, ability and experience of both the surgeon and the anaesthetist, and degree of discomfort both prior to and postoperatively. The risk of anaesthesia can be graded according to the American Society of Anaesthesiologists (ASA) risk assessment listed in Table 6.2. Preoperative blood tests or fluid therapy might be appropriate at this stage. If the animal is calm, an intravenous catheter can be placed now, although sometimes it is left until after the premedication has taken effect, especially in the face of potential globe rupture, such as with a very deep corneal ulcer where it is vital that the animal does not struggle and risk the ulcer perforating. During this

Table 6.2 American Society of Anaesthesiologists (ASA) risk assessment

Grade	Description
1	Healthy patient
2	Mild systemic disease, no functional limitation
3	Severe systemic disease, definite functional limitation but not incapacitating
4	Severe systemic disease that is a constant threat to life
5	Moribund patient, unlikely to survive 24 hours, with or without surgery
E	An E is placed after the appropriate grade if the patient is presented on an emergency basis—for example, a corneal foreign body where the recommended preoperative procedures such as withholding food might not have occurred

Reproduced with permission from the American Society of Anesthesiologists, 520 N. Northwest Highway, Park Ridge, Illinois 60068–2573

period, the preparation area should be cleaned and made ready, and all equipment thoroughly checked.

2. Pre-anaesthetic period

The pre-anaesthetic medication (premed) is given. This is usually a combination of sedative and analgesic, and will reduce anxiety and relive discomfort. As part of a balanced anaesthetic protocol, this allows lower levels of induction and maintenance agents to be used. The animal should be left quiet and undisturbed for the medication to take effect, although it should be closely observed.

3. Induction period

If an intravenous catheter has not been placed already it is placed now. This allows easy administration of intravenous agents and prevents the risk of extravascular spillage. It also provides instant access to the vascular system should an emergency arise. Suitable endotracheal tubes, anaesthetic breathing circuits and monitoring equipment are prepared prior to the administration of the anaesthetic induction agent. Intravenous fluids should be set up if required during the surgery.

4. Maintenance period

The animal is kept unconscious with the use of inhalational or injectable drugs. Every patient should

have an anaesthetic record sheet which must be properly completed (Fig. 6.1).

5. Recovery period

The anaesthetic agents are stopped and the animal is allowed to regain consciousness. Oxygen therapy should be continued as the animal begins to wake up. The patient must be closely monitored until fully recovered. The intravenous catheter should not be removed until the animal is fully conscious.

Consent for anaesthesia

The nurse is often delegated to obtain written consent for anaesthesia from the client, and it should be remembered that it is a legal requirement to obtain such informed consent. An example consent form is shown in Figure 6.2. The veterinary surgeon in charge of the case should have fully explained the procedure to be undertaken, but it is always sensible for the nurse to repeat this. Sometimes owners will be more inclined to ask questions or express concerns to the nurse rather than the veterinary surgeon. The risks of the anaesthetic, together with those of the procedure, should be fully explained, while at the same time reassuring the client. The time that the animal last ate and drank should be recorded. For elective procedures, fasting for at least 6–8 hours is recommended. Water is usually only withheld once the premedication

Date: 　　　Name: 　　　Owner:

Weight: 　　　Sex: 　　　Breed:

Operation: 　　　Age: 　　　Rate:

VS: 　　　Anaesthetist:

Pre-op Preparation:

Pre-med				E	G	F	P	VP
1		4						
2		5		Time				
3				Effect				

ET Tube = 　　　Pulse oximeter = 　　　Blood Pressure =

Circuit = 　　　Oesophageal stethoscope = 　　　Capillary refill time =

Oesophageal Thermometer = 　　　ECG = 　　　Mucous membranes colour =

Drugs given

NOTES

1 mg																							
2 mg																							
3 isofluorane %																							
4 Oxygen L/Min																							
Temperature																							
240																							
230																							
220																							

Code:

Pulse = ●

Fig. 6.1 Anaesthesia record sheet.

		210																			
Resp = **o**		210																			
		200																			
Ventilate = ∅		190																			
		180																			
Pulse		170																			
Oximeter = **P**		160																			
		150																			
CRT = [sec]		140																			
∆		130																			
MM = colour		120																			
		110																			
B Pressure		100																			
Systolic = **V**		90																			
Diastolic = ∧		80																			
		70																			
		60																			
		50																			
		40																			
		30																			
		20																			
		10																			

Recovery

Fluid Therapy

Catheter =

Fluid =

Rate of infusion =

Volume of fluid =

Blood Loss =

Time of drugs and notes

Copyright SueMothersdale.VN Dip AVN[surg]

Fig. 6.1 Anaesthesia record sheet—*continued.*

FORM OF CONSENT

Patient Details: Name _____

Breed/Description _____

Colour _____ Sex _____ Age _____

Starved: YES/NO   Water: YES/NO   Vaccinated: YES/NO   **Your Pet is at risk if vaccinations are not up to date**

Pulse/Respiration: _____ Weight: _____

Known Allergies: _____ Current Medication: _____

Owner's Details: Name: _____

Address: _____

Tel: Home _____ Work _____

Mobile _____ Other _____

Procedures To Be Performed: Full General Anaesthesia / Sedation + _____
                              (Delete as appropriate)

I hereby give my permission for .... Veterinary Centre to administer an anaesthetic or sedation to the above animal and to perform the above procedure and any additional diagnostic and/or treatment procedures as deemed necessary for my pet. The procedures have been explained to me and I understand that, as with all anaesthetic techniques and surgical procedures, there is a risk involved.

In order to minimize the risks we will perform a full physical examination on your pet. However, we highly recommend a pre-surgical blood test to eliminate the possibility of pre-existing problems that may not be evident on physical examination but which could lead to complications during or following anaesthesia. This is particularly important in older animals (those aged seven or over).

I do/do not wish the pre-surgical blood test to be performed.

Estimate of Cost £_____exc VAT. I understand that estimates are not a guarantee of the final cost of treatment for my pet. I understand that ………….. veterinary centre reserves the right to exceed the above estimate by as much as 20% without prior consultation and that by signing below I am agreeing to meet these costs. I also understand that treatment likely to exceed this 20% margin will be cleared with me in advance.

I have read, understood and agreed to the above. I am aware that I must settle the account in full prior to release of the above named pet and by signing this form I agree to accept financial responsibility for the treatment given.

Signature of owner or agent: _____ **Date:** _____

Name of owner or agent: _____ **Please Print Clearly**

Note: Admitted with pet were Basket/Lead/Collar/Toys/Blanket.   Such items are at owners risk and the veterinary centre will accept no responsibility for damage or loss. It is recommended that any such items be taken home.

          Owner Contacted at: _____By:_____

Fig. 6.2 Consent form for anaesthesia and surgery.

agents have been given. Only once the owners are happy that their animal will be carefully looked after, and that all steps will be taken to reduce the risks involved, should they be asked to sign the consent form. In addition to signing and dating the form, all contact numbers should be double-checked (with an indication of which is the best number to try first if more than one contact number is supplied) and a note made of any concurrent medical conditions (e.g. diabetes mellitus) and any medication the animal is receiving (both ocular and general). If the owner leaves any belongings with their pet, these should be labelled and listed on the consent form.

Health and safety aspects

For details of health and safety legislation, refer to the bibliography at the end of this chapter. Several regulations are enforced to minimise the risk of exposure to hazardous substances and to limit accidents. These include general health and safety, substances hazardous to health and the misuse of drugs. Specific hazards, such as compressed gas cylinders and exposure to volatile anaesthetics, are also covered. General personnel safety must also be considered (e.g. sharps disposal, care when lifting patients, etc.).

PHYSIOLOGY AND ANAESTHESIA

In addition to the general aspects of physiology as it relates to anaesthesia, there are several specific points which need to be considered with regard to ophthalmic procedures. Factors such as respiratory, cardiovascular, renal, hepatic and nervous system effects are discussed in specific textbooks about anaesthesia (see Bibliography). For example, the effect of positioning on ventilation and perfusion, acid–base balance, blood pressure effects, renal excretion and blood flow during anaesthesia, along with drug transportation and metabolism via hepatic routes must all be considered. Detailed discussion of these is beyond the scope of this text but, nonetheless, nurses should be familiar with them.

The principal aspects of ocular physiology which need to be considered are intraocular pressure effects and the oculocardiac reflex.

Intraocular pressure effects

Intraocular pressure is determined by the balance between the production and removal of aqueous humour, together with the volume of vitreous humour, the blood volume within the uveal vascular system and the extraocular muscle tone. Thus, there are many factors to consider. Sudden alterations in intraocular pressure can have severe consequences. For example, a sudden increase can compromise retinal blood flow, causing retinal degeneration and blindness to develop, or can induce vitreous prolapse during surgery. Intraocular pressure is influenced by venous pressure, direct pressure on the globe, endotracheal intubation, ventilation, systemic blood pressure and various drugs.

Elevations in venous pressure will cause a rise in intraocular pressure. Things which can increase venous pressure include compression of the jugular veins during the collection of a blood sample, a collar around the neck (thus a harness or lead across the chest is preferred, as shown in Fig. 4.3, p. 56), and inappropriate positioning for surgery. Airway obstruction will lead to a rapid increase in venous pressure, and thus armoured endotracheal tubes should be considered for procedures which require flexion of the neck. Vomiting will raise intraocular pressure and, therefore, agents which can induce this must be avoided for pre-medication (morphine, xylazine and medetomidine should be avoided if intraocular pressure elevation is of concern). Coughing has the same effect as vomiting in raising intraocular pressure and should also be avoided. The patient must be in a sufficient plane of anaesthesia for endotracheal intubation; if too light, then coughing might occur.

Direct pressure on the globe will increase intraocular pressure. Thus, if face masks are used they should be carefully placed so as not to touch the eyes. Care should also be taken when positioning the patient so as not to put pressure on either eye—the non-surgical or 'down side' eye is particularly at risk.

As mentioned above, endotracheal intubation can affect intraocular pressure if performed under a light plane of anaesthesia, as it can induce coughing. In addition, blood pressure and laryngeal reflexes are altered during intubation, and deleterious effects on these can be minimised by touching the larynx as little as possible during the intubation process. The use of a lignocaine spray on the larynx prior to intubation is recommended, especially in cats. Particular care must also be taken during intubation if the globe has ruptured or may rupture—clearly a sudden rise in intraocular pressure in these circumstances would be a disaster.

Blood pressure can affect intraocular pressure. Although intraocular pressure is normally stable over a wide range of systemic blood pressure values, any sudden rise, such as during a painful surgical stimulus, can increase intraocular pressure. In addition, the animal's ability to autoregulate intraocular pressure might be reduced during anaesthesia. Thus, a suitable plane of anaesthesia, together with appropriate analgesia and regular blood pressure monitoring, should avoid this potential problem. Good ventilation must also be ensured since this will have a direct affect on blood flow in the ocular vessels. For example, hypercapnia will cause vasodilation, and this can raise intraocular pressure. Careful monitoring is essential (p. 96).

One final factor to consider in discussing intraocular pressure is the effect of drugs. Commonly used agents for premedication such as acetylpromazine and benzodiazepines either cause a slight decrease in intraocular pressure or no effect at all. Opioids are similar unless vomiting occurs. The choice of agents for anaesthesia is discussed later in this chapter (from p. 90). Concurrent medication, either ophthalmic or for other problems, might need consideration. This is mentioned later in the section on patient preparation, but an example could be a patient receiving a topical adrenergic agonist such as phenylephrine. This could increase systemic blood pressure which might elevate intraocular pressure.

Oculocardiac reflex

The oculocardiac reflex is a second important aspect of ocular physiology to be aware of when considering anaesthesia. This reflex occurs when a stimulus to the eye (which could be surgical manipulation, traction or pressure) is transmitted centrally though the trigeminal nerve (cranial nerve V) where it connects to the vagus nerve (cranial nerve X) (Fig. 6.3). This can result in a profound bradycardia, arrhythmias and even asystole. Although less of a concern in dogs and cats than in people, it is still a risk and one must be alerted to the possibility of its occurrence should the heart rate suddenly drop during surgery. If ignored, cardiac arrest and death can occur. The use of atropine intravenously (0.02 mg/kg) together with cessation of the stimulus should reverse the effect.

PREOPERATIVE ASSESSMENT

Careful preoperative evaluation of the patient is as important with ophthalmic surgery as for any other procedure. It is necessary to identify physiological, pathological and drug-related factors which could affect both the anaesthetic and the procedure to be undertaken.

A detailed history must be obtained from the owner. The patient should be assessed with reference to:

- age, breed, sex
- whether neutered

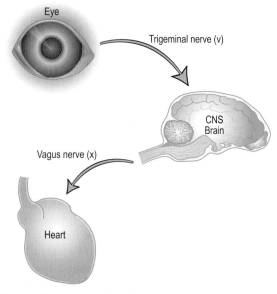

Fig. 6.3 The oculocardiac reflex.

- previous anaesthesia and response to it
- concurrent drug therapy (both ophthalmic and for other disease).

A full clinical examination must be undertaken, and baseline temperature, pulse and respiration rates recorded. Patients for ocular surgery can be very young (e.g. prolapsed nictitans glands at 12 weeks of age in an English bulldog) or old (e.g. 13-year-old collie needing cataract surgery). Elective surgery in elderly or geriatric patients (the latter are defined as those older than 75–80% of their expected life span) is not uncommon in ophthalmic practice. In addition to any concurrent disease, these patients can be expected to have decreased rates of drug elimination and to require lower amounts of premedicants and induction agents simply as a result of age changes. They may have decreased renal perfusion and lowered oxygenation levels which need addressing. Preoperative blood tests would normally be undertaken in older patients and those with known medical conditions, such as diabetes mellitus or cardiac disease. Intravenous fluid therapy might be started in the preoperative phase to achieve safe, balanced anaesthesia.

Concurrent medication commonly encountered in ophthalmic patients might include systemic non-steroidal anti-inflammatory drugs (NSAIDs) for arthritis, ACE-inhibitors for cardiac disease, or corticosteroids for atopic conditions. These can affect the choice of drugs for anaesthesia.

Catheter placement

It is good nursing practice to always place an intravenous catheter prior to general anaesthesia. For ophthalmic patients it is sometimes preferable to use the saphenous vein rather than the cephalic for ease of access during surgery (Fig. 6.4). Remember that the head will be fully draped and thus access to the front legs can be limited.

Pain assessment

Pain must be assessed and adequately managed prior to, during and after anaesthesia. Pain is detri-

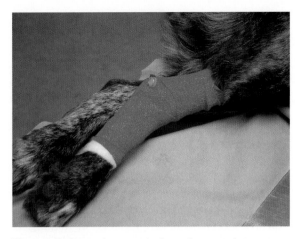

Fig. 6.4 Catheter placement in the saphenous vein.

mental to animals undergoing anaesthesia and surgery. It may cause an animal to hypoventilate, leading to hypoxia, hypercapnia and acidosis; it also prolongs anaesthetic recovery and reduces cardiovascular function among several other effects. Behavioural assessment can be both a practical and sensitive measurement of pain. This is discussed in detail elsewhere (p. 57), but certain factors are particularly relevant in respect to eye problems. Vocalisation (whining, whimpering, howling, hissing, etc.) should be avoided since it can increase intraocular pressure. Remember that many animals will become particularly quiet if in pain. Abnormal posture, particularly head pressing against the kennel walls, is a sign of discomfort which can damage the eye. Self mutilation with attempts at rubbing the sore eye should be prevented; adequate analgesia will often achieve this without the need for Elizabethan collars. How the animal responds to interaction with nurses, including how it reacts to having the eye cleaned or medication applied, will give an indication of whether or not it is in discomfort.

The use of an analgesic prior to inflicting pain (a surgical procedure in this case) will produce better pain control than just using an analgesic agent after the event, and as such analgesic drugs are usually included with the premed. An exception to this could be if the animal is already receiving such agents orally to treat the pain associated with their condition and are not due another dose of analgesic at the time of surgery.

Handling the ophthalmic patient

As mentioned above, it is important to avoid increases in intraocular pressure in certain patients. These include glaucoma patients, but also those with deep corneal ulcers or foreign bodies where a sudden rise in pressure could result in disastrous globe rupture. The use of a harness or lead around the chest rather than a collar has been mentioned already. For the same reason, blood samples might be best taken from the cephalic rather than the jugular veins. Patients for ocular surgery might be blind and thus require special consideration—for example, lots of talking to and reassuring, keeping on a short lead for dogs and minimal movement about the clinic. This is discussed in more detail in Chapter 4.

ANAESTHETIC PLAN

The process of anaesthesia is divided into the five stages, as listed at the beginning of this chapter (namely preoperative, pre-anaesthetic (premed), induction, maintenance and recovery periods). An outline plan should be drawn up considering the choice of drugs, breathing circuit, monitoring equipment and recovery needs of the patient.

Fluid therapy

Patients undergoing anaesthesia for ophthalmic surgery might require fluid therapy to provide circulatory support and to replace fluid losses. Anaesthetised patients can lose more fluids than conscious patients, through drug effects, increased respiratory loss, evaporation from the surgical site (minimal in ocular surgery) and blood loss (again minimal with the exception of some enucleation procedures). The choice of infusion agent varies according to the patient's needs, but in most cases an isotonic balanced crystalloid such as Hartmann's solution/lactated Ringer's is appropriate. The rate of infusion will depend on the rate of loss, health of the patient, type of fluid and response to fluid therapy. An infusion pump is advised to provide accurate fluid replacement. This is particularly important in small patients (e.g. cats), where over-perfusion can easily occur.

Mannitol is sometimes used preoperatively to lower intraocular pressure. This can make some types of surgery (e.g. removing anterior lens luxation) easier with the reduced risk of both intra- and postoperative complication. Renal function should be checked prior to its use, and it may cause potential anaesthetic problems by increasing plasma osmolarity, circulating blood volume and central venous pressure.

ANAESTHETIC DRUGS

We will divide anaesthetic drugs into those used for premedication, induction and maintenance. There is some overlap between these groups—for example, propofol can be used for both induction and maintenance.

Premedication

The objectives of premedication are as follows:
- to calm the patient and reduce anxiety prior to induction of anaesthesia
- to provide sedation
- to aid with smooth induction and recovery
- to reduce the levels of induction and maintenance agents required
- to provide analgesia
- to reduce any side-effects of other anaesthetic agents
- to reduce the adverse effects of surgery.

A calm, sedated patient is less likely to struggle during handling and induction. This will reduce the risk of ocular damage (such as might be incurred as the animal struggles on the table) and will minimise increases in intraocular pressure. The importance of a smooth induction cannot be overemphasised for ocular procedures. Levels of induction and maintenance agents can be reduced by 30–50% by the use of a suitable premedication. If the animal has shown signs of pain, it might have already received some form of analgesia. This should be 'topped up', or a different class of drug included (e.g. an opioid if the animal is already on NSAIDs). The pre-emptive use of analgesics as part of a balanced anaesthetic regime is to be encouraged. Postoperative pain management is easier if the patient has received analgesia prior to surgery. The premedication will often last longer than the surgery, and as such will allow a smooth recovery as well. For ocular procedures this is vital since any coughing, retching, or excessive attempts at moving while still uncoordinated could have catastrophic consequences on the delicate surgery.

Sufficient time must pass between the administration of the premedication and induction. This will vary according to the agents given and the route of administration.

The commonly used premedicants in ophthalmic anaesthesia are the phenothiazines, together with opioids. Benzodiazepines are also used. Alpha-2-adrenoceptor agonists are occasionally used, as are antimuscarinics.

Phenothiazines are routinely used as part of a premedication, and acepromazine (ACP) is usually chosen. It is available as a solution of 2 mg/ml and is given at doses ranging from 0.01–0.05 mg/kg. It can be given by subcutaneous, intramuscular or intravenous routes. It lasts for 4–6 hours but is slow in onset, taking 20–30 minutes. Given in conjunction with an opioid it has improved sedative effects. In addition, it has antiemetic and antiarrythmic effects, but disadvantages include hypotension, unpredictability (e.g. aggressive dogs are often resistant to its effects) and hypothermia. It has no analgesic effect. Care must be taken in epileptics, as it reduces the seizure threshold, and in certain breeds (e.g. boxer), where syncope can occur.

By using ACP in combination with an opioid (neuroleptanalgesia), good reliable sedation is achieved along with analgesia at relatively modest dose rates. Side-effects on cardiovascular and respiratory systems are mild. Opioids reduce the requirements of induction and maintenance agents (this applies even when administered on their own). They are useful in ophthalmic surgery for their antitussive effect—they suppress coughing which can be detrimental pre- and post-surgery by raising intraocular pressure. Some opioids do cause vomiting (e.g. morphine), so these are best avoided in favour of similar drugs, such as methadone. The choice of opioid will also depend on the degree of pain anticipated. More potent drugs (pure agonists), such as methadone, should be chosen over 'weaker' agents, such as buprenorphine (partial agonist), if severe pain is anticipated. In

the UK, most opioids are controlled drugs and subject to specific legislation (Misuse of Drugs Act 1971). This affects their use and storage.

Methadone (0.1–0.5 mg/kg for dogs; 0.1–0.2 mg/kg for cats) is usually given by intramuscular injection and its effects last about 4 hours. Morphine is similar. Pethidine (1.0–5.0 mg/kg in dogs or cats) is also used but has a shorter duration of action of only about 2 hours. These three agents are pure agonists and as such have a dose dependent effect—higher or repeated doses will have greater analgesic effect. Bupernorphine is widely used in veterinary anaesthesia. It is a partial agonist, rather than a pure agonist, and cannot be used in conjunction with a pure opioid. It has an unusual bell-shaped response curve, which means that it may achieve less analgesia at high doses or if topped-up frequently. Thus, it is generally used only where mild or moderate pain is anticipated. Doses of 0.006–0.02 mg/kg are given, usually by intramuscular route. It has a slow onset of action (45 minutes) but long duration of action (6–8 hours). Butorphanol is another opioid which provides inconsistent analgesia, but its antitussive properties mean that it is occasionally chosen for ophthalmic use.

Benzodiazepines produce mild muscle relaxation, reduce anxiety, provide amnesia and hypnosis, and have some sedative-like effects. They are very useful in epileptic patients, as they have powerful anticonvulsant effects. They have a wide safety margin and enhance the effects of other general anaesthetic agents. They provide a good choice for debilitated animals. However, they can be unpredictable in healthy animals and can cause excitement. Diazepam can be painful on injection when given by both intramuscular and intravenous routes. Despite this, it is most commonly administered by intramuscular injection. However, giving the agent by slow intravenous injection results in less discomfort. Alternatively, a water-soluble emulsion of diazepam (Diazemuls, Dumex) or a slightly different drug such as midazolam (Hyponvel, Roche) can be used since neither of these agents are painful when injected. For both diazepam and midazolam, doses of 0.1–0.2 mg/kg are usually given.

Alpha-2-adrenoceptor agonists are potent sedatives which also provide some analgesia and muscle relaxation. However, they cause profound cardiopulmonary depression at moderate and higher doses and should not be used in debilitated patients without good reason. An advantage is that they have specific antagonists which rapidly reverse their action. The duration of action is dose dependent, and they do allow for a dramatic reduction in the amounts of induction and maintenance agents required. Vomiting can be triggered, especially with xylazine (Rompun, Bayer) and this agent should be used with care in ophthalmic patients. Medetomidine (Domitor, Pfizer) is more commonly used and should be administered at the lower end of the range (10–20 μ/kg). If used for more profound sedation rather than as a premedication, higher doses can be administered (see p. 100 for discussion on sedation for minor procedures). Atipamezole (Antisedan, Pfizer) is used to antagonise and, thereby, reverse the medetomidine. It reverses the analgesic, as well as the sedative, effects of the agonist, and a suitable analgesic should be given if not already administered. Some animals are easily roused while under alpha-2-agonist sedation; they are often noise sensitive, for example, and caution should be exercised to avoid sudden noises if patients are premedicated with alpha-2-adrenoceptors.

Anticholinergic (antimuscarinic) agents can be used if required as part of a premedication, but are not usually necessary with the advent of modern volatile anaesthetics. Some anaesthetists are in favour of their routine use, while others feel they are largely unnecessary. Individual preference will vary tremendously. Anticholinergic agents decrease salivation and bronchial secretion (useful in small patients such as cats where endotracheal tubes can easily block with secretions) and protect against unwanted effects of certain drugs—most commonly the adverse vagal effects of anticholinesterase drugs which are used to reverse neuromuscular blocks (see below). They can also be used to protect against and treat vagally induced bradycardia (e.g. oculocardiac reflex). Potential disadvantages include increased metabolic rate, increased heart rate and oxygen consumption, gastrointestinal ileus (especially in horses), pupil dilation and visual disturbance. The latter is more common in cats and can occasionally cause them to panic on recovery. The pupil dilation can trigger glaucoma in predisposed animals, and anticholinergic agents should be avoided in such situations. Atropine is most commonly used at doses of 0.02–0.04 mg/kg by intramuscular, subcutaneous or slow intravenous injection. Glycopyrrolate (0.01–0.02 mg/kg) is less commonly used.

Analgesia

As mentioned in previous sections, the use of an analgesic in combination with a sedative is a preferred basis for premedication. Prevention of pain will provide a more stable anaesthetic and better recovery from surgery. In addition to the opioids discussed above, NSAIDs and local anaesthetics can be used. Carprofen (Rimadyl, Pfizer) at a dose of 4 mg/kg by subcutaneous or intravenous injection in both dogs and cats and meloxicam (Metacam, Boehringer Ingleheim) at a dose of 0.2 mg/kg in dogs and 0.3 mg/kg in cats by subcutaneous injection, are currently the most widely used NSAIDs. Other agents include aspirin, ketoprofen and flunixin, but these are less commonly used. All NSAIDs can affect platelet function, renal perfusion and cause some gastric irritation to variable degrees, depending on each drug. Carprofen exhibits potent anti-inflammatory and analgesic effects, and (along with meloxicam) can be used preoperatively as part of the balanced approach to anaesthesia, with pre-emptive analgesia providing maximal benefit.

Local anaesthetics block pain perception peripherally so that the noxious insult does not get transmitted to the CNS. Topical proxymetacaine can be used alone or in conjunction with sedation for minor procedures, such as the debridement of an ulcer or a conjunctival biopsy. It is occasionally used as part of the array of topical agents applied prior to intraocular surgery, as it provides good local anaesthesia. However, it is toxic to corneal epithelial cells and can delay wound healing, so is not recommended for frequent use.

Local infiltration of anaesthetic agents such as lignocaine can be used to block regional nerves (e.g. retrobulbar blocks or auriculopalpebral blocks). These are usually reserved for farm species and horses where surgery can be performed in the standing animal. They are mentioned in the section on equine anaesthesia later in this chapter.

Induction

The induction of anaesthesia is usually achieved via an intravenous injection, although intramuscular injections and occasionally inhalational agents can be used. The latter ('masking down') are not recommended for ophthalmic procedures since they can be extremely distressing for the patient, leading to increases in blood pressure and intraocular pressure with potential damage to the eyes.

Propofol is the induction agent of choice for most ophthalmic procedures. It has a quick onset and smooth, rapid recovery. A suitable premedication must always be given for ophthalmic procedures, since the rapid recovery could lead to excitement or trauma in the unsedated patient. Dose rates vary from 3–8 mg/kg. The drug is rapidly metabolised, mainly in the liver. It can be used as a maintenance agent as well, by incremental top-up injections or constant infusion. It does cause some cardiovascular and respiratory depression at similar levels to thiopental (thiopentone), and occasionally post-induction apnoea is encountered with propofol. Since the emulsion of drug supports bacterial growth, opened ampoules or multidose vials should be discarded after 8 hours.

Thiopental is a barbiturate drug which causes a rapid-onset anaesthesia. It causes hypotension and sensitises the heart to catecholamines (arrhythmias can be seen on induction). It causes a dose-dependent respiratory depression (thus endotracheal intubation is essential). It should be administered via an intravenous catheter since any extravascular spillage is irritating and can cause skin sloughing. Once the powder has been reconstituted with sterile water, it should be discarded after 24 hours since the solution is not stable. A dose rate of 10 mg/kg is standard but will vary according to the premed received and the health of the patient. Recovery from anaesthesia is via redistribution of the drug through body tissues (especially adipose tissue) and sight-hounds and thin animals experience a delayed recovery with prolonged hangover period. The longer recovery seen with thiopental versus propofol can cause animals to be confused and ataxic, and inadvertently damage their eyes as they struggle to get up.

'Saffan' is a steroid mixture used for induction and maintenance of anaesthesia in cats (given by intramuscular or intravenous injection). Although it causes a smooth induction with minimal respiratory depression, recovery is often very excitable and it is not recommended for ophthalmic procedures.

Ketamine produces a dissociative anaesthesia (light sleep with good analgesia and amnesia). Eyelid and corneal reflexes remain intact, and the eyes stay open (lubrication for the non-operated eye is mandatory). It should not be used as a sole induction agent, as seizures can occur especially in dogs. For this reason it is typically combined with an alpha-2-agonist or a benzodiazepine. Increases in blood pressure can affect intraocular pressure, which is not recommended for eye surgery. Increased muscle tone in the extraocular muscles can also raise the intraocular pressure. Ketamine must not be used in eyes which are perforated, or might become so (e.g. deep corneal ulcer), for these same reasons.

Maintenance

Once induction of anaesthesia has been achieved, endotracheal intubation should be performed for all eye surgery, even if intravenous agents such as propofol are used for maintenance. Total intravenous anaesthesia is rarely used for ophthalmic surgery and will not be discussed further.

Endotracheal intubation ensures a patent airway and prevents aspiration of fluids or regurgitated food. Cuffed tubes are more commonly used in ocular surgery, especially if any oral involvement might occur, for example during parotid duct transposition or for the investigation of retrobulbar abscesses. Cuffed tubes are essential if neuromuscular-blocking drugs and positive-pressure ventilation are used. Since positioning for ocular surgery can result in marked flexion of the neck, armoured tubes might be advisable as these will not kink or occlude with positioning (Fig. 6.5). It is important to ensure adequate induction prior to intubation—the animal must not gag or cough. In cats it is essential to desensitise the larynx with a local anaesthetic spray prior to attempting intubation. The tube should be tied in place. Often it is necessary to tie to the lower jaw, rather than the upper jaw or behind the head; the latter two

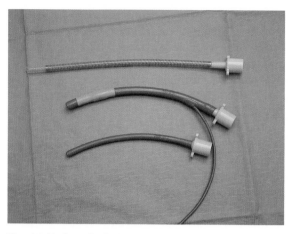

Fig. 6.5 Endotracheal tubes—armoured, cuffed and uncuffed (top to bottom).

positions may get in the way of the surgical field (Fig. 6.6). At the end of surgery, animals should be extubated before the gag reflex fully returns so they are less likely to cough and cause damage to the surgical site.

Details of anaesthetic machines and breathing circuits are beyond the scope of this book (see the bibliography at the end of this chapter for further information if required). Suffice to say that all equipment must be switched on and checked prior to use. Various factors will influence the choice of machine and circuit, such as the size of animal, whether intermittent positive pressure ventilation

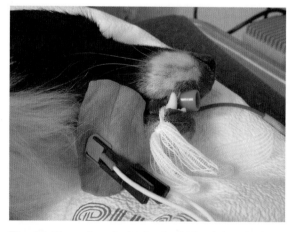

Fig. 6.6 The endotracheal tube should be tied to the lower jaw so that it does not get in the way of the surgeon (also note pulse oximeter on tongue).

will be required, whether nitrous oxide is being used and the anticipated length of time the procedure will take.

Inhalational agents are usually used for maintenance of anaesthesia, and the most frequently encountered are isoflurane and halothane in a mixture with oxygen. Further details of the pharmacokinetics of many of these agents can be found in the sources listed in the bibliography at the end of this chapter. The rate of onset and recovery from inhalational anaesthesia depends on many factors including the concentration of anaesthetic agent used, the alveolar ventilation (e.g. hyperventilation leads to more rapid uptake of the gaseous anaesthetic while hypoventilation will slow uptake and elimination of the anaesthetic), the blood:gas solubility of the agent, the blood:tissue solubility and the cardiac output of the patient. In general, inhalational agents are eliminated by exhalation, although there is some metabolism by the body. Table 6.3 details ideal characteristics of an inhalational agent.

Isoflurane has now overtaken halothane as the inhalational agent of choice for veterinary surgery and is recommended for ophthalmic surgery. Uptake and elimination is faster than for halothane, and depth of anaesthesia can be more easily altered. Isoflurane allows a more stable cardiac rhythm than halothane because it does not sensitise the heart to catecholamines (i.e. adrenaline). It also provides better muscle relaxation (including extraocular muscles). Some arterial hypotension is caused by both isoflurane and halothane, and this means that they are both safe to use in glaucomatous patients. Halothane may lead to bradycardia, and this should be borne in mind during ocular surgery where the oculocardiac reflex (see above) could slow the heart further. Newer agents, such as sevoflurane, are becoming more widely used. Sevoflurane allows even more rapid control of anaesthetic depth (and has been advocated for 'masking down' since its effects are so rapid). However, this method of induction is still is not advised for ophthalmic surgery.

Nitrous oxide is a very weak anaesthetic and must be combined with isoflurane or halothane. It will lower the percentage of these agents required to maintain the same level of anaesthesia than if used without nitrous oxide. Another advantage of nitrous oxide is the fact that it has some analgesic properties. One potential disadvantage with

Table 6.3 The ideal properties of an inhalational anaesthetic agent

Agent properties	Action on patient
• Easily vaporised • Non-toxic • Non-flammable and non-explosive • Stable on storage • Low blood:gas solubility • Mean alveolar concentration low enough to allow delivery with high oxygen concentrations • Compatible with soda lime	• Good analgesic • Non irritant to mucous membranes • Little effect on respiratory and cardiovascular function • Good muscle relaxation • Minimal or no body metabolism of agent • Rapid uptake and smooth induction of anaesthesia • Rapid elimination and smooth recovery from anaesthesia

regard to ophthalmic use is the fact that it diffuses rapidly into any body gas pockets, resulting in the expansion of the gas pocket. Air is sometimes injected into eyes to help to reinflate them following intraocular surgery (e.g. removal of an anterior lens luxation). Expansion of this could lead to increased intraocular pressure, including overt glaucoma, and would put undue pressure on the suture line. Thus, communication between surgeon and anaesthetist is mandatory if this type of surgery is being undertaken with the use of nitrous oxide.

Muscle relaxant anaesthesia

Neuromuscular blocking agents (muscle relaxants) are commonly used in ophthalmic surgery. Advantages of muscle relaxant anaesthesia for ocular surgery include guaranteed immobility—for microsurgery this is essential. The eye position is maintained centrally (no rolling down), which makes access to the cornea and intraocular structures much easier. The extraocular muscles are totally relaxed, such that no pressure is exerted on the posterior globe and thereby the vitreous. This reduces the risk of complications such as forward prolapse of the vitreous during cataract surgery.

These drugs work at the neuromuscular junction of all skeletal muscle (including the respiratory muscles of the intercostals and diaphragm) but do not affect cardiac or smooth muscle. Supported ventilation, usually with a ventilator, is required, although on occasions manual intermittent positive pressure ventilation (IPPV) is used. Neuromuscular blocking agents do not cross the blood–brain barrier and thus have no effect on consciousness,

but they do prevent some signs of inadequate anaesthesia, such as movement and eye position. Therefore, the anaesthetist has to be vigilant in monitoring to ensure that the animal is properly unconscious and pain-free. Signs which could suggest inadequate anaesthesia include mydriasis and lacrimation (difficult to assess during ocular procedures as the pupil is often pharmacologically dilated and the eye is flushed with balanced salt solution), salivation, tachycardia, hypertension and increased end-tidal CO_2 levels. A peripheral nerve stimulator can also be used to measure the degree of relaxation but gives no indications about anaesthetic depth. The most common pattern of peripheral nerve stimulation is the train of four (TOF) applied by electrodes attached over a peripheral nerve, such as the ulnar or peroneal nerve (lateral tibia, usually more easy to access during ocular surgery). A normal animal with no relaxant will have four equal twitches in the TOF, while 'fade' will occur under muscle relaxant such that each subsequent twitch is smaller than the previous one. Usually only one or two of the four twitches remain during ideal muscle relaxation.

Ventilation during muscle relaxant anaesthesia is best achieved using a mechanical ventilator which is set to the requirements of the individual patient (Fig. 6.7). Ventilators are usually pressure, volume or time-cycled, each with advantages and disadvantages. Mechanical ventilation is safer than long-term manual ventilation and frees up the anaesthetist to monitor effectively. All artificial ventilation can have profound and complicated effects on respiratory and cardiovascular physiology (discussion of which are beyond the scope of this book), and these effects can alter the course of the anaes-

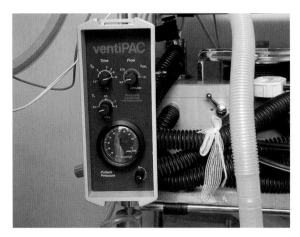

Fig. 6.7 Ventilator.

thetic. Due to these facts, along with the complexity of assessing the degree of anaesthesia, reversing the blockade (see below) and deciding when the patient can safely breathe spontaneously, it is suggested that this type of anaesthetic should only be given by a veterinary anaesthetist or a very experienced nurse under direct supervision of an anaesthetist.

Table 6.4 lists the signs of inadequate anaesthesia during neuromuscular blockade.

The most commonly used muscle relaxants are the non-depolarising types, with pancuronium, vecuronium and atacurium being the most widely used. They are given intravenously. None are licensed for veterinary use. Generally, they last 20–40 minutes, depending on the agent used, and

can be topped up if longer surgery time occurs. Length of efficacy may vary considerably between individuals. Atacurium has a rapid onset of action and can be used in animals with renal or hepatic disease since it is spontaneously degraded without the need for body metabolism.

Non-depolarising muscle relaxants can be reversed with anticholinesterases—usually neostigmine, although edrophonium is sometimes used. Ventilation must be maintained until adequate spontaneous respiration occurs. Anticholinergic (antimuscarinic) drugs are often required along with the anticholinesterase to reduce the bradycardia, salivation, bronchospasm and defecation seen alongside the reversal of blockade. The TOF can be monitored to evaluate the return of four full twitches following reversal. In addition to removing the blockade, the animal must be woken from anaesthesia. If anaesthesia is too 'deep' on administration of the reversal agent, the return of spontaneous respiration will be delayed. This is potentially a critical time for the patient.

Monitoring

Careful and frequent monitoring during anaesthesia allows rapid intervention if changes in the patient are detected. This ensures patient safety. In addition to providing an appropriate depth of anaesthesia, monitoring facilitates the maintenance of near-normal physiological function—cardiovascu-

Table 6.4 Signs of inadequate anaesthesia during muscle relaxation
Signs of inadequate anaesthesia during muscle relaxation
• Increase in arterial blood pressure
• Increased heart rate
• Salivation
• Increased tear production (not usually visible during eye surgery where frequent irrigation is used)
• Signs of vagovagal syncope—bradycardia, pallor, hypotension
• Increased end-tidal CO_2
• Slight twitching of face or tongue (again not usually appreciated during eye surgery as this region is fully draped)
Signs which cannot be assessed due to the neuromuscular agent
• The eye is central anyway so will not rotate up
• The eyelids are paralysed so no palpebral (blink reflex) can occur
• The animal will not move or have a pedal withdrawal reflex
• Respiratory rate will not increase since the muscles are paralysed

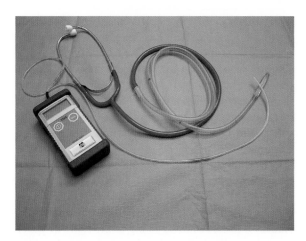

Fig. 6.8 Oesophageal stethoscope and oesophageal thermometer.

lar, respiratory and body temperature control. A written record (Fig. 6.1) should be completed for each patient, with recordings taken at least every 5 minutes. Several of the parameters normally used to assess depth of anaesthesia cannot be used in ophthalmic surgery, as they are at the surgical site. Thus the palpebral (blink) reflex, eye position, pupil size, lacrimation, jaw tone, tongue curl and salivation cannot be properly assessed. One has to rely on respiratory signs (the rate, depth and pattern of breathing), cardiovascular signs (heart rate, blood pressure, rate and quality of peripheral pulses) and anaesthetic depth and muscle tone with the response to a toe pinch. The dorsal pedal artery is usually used to assess rate, rhythm and quality of the peripheral pulse since it will be more easily accessible than the metacarpal artery. Capillary refill time cannot be easily assessed from the gum, as is usual, so another site such as the vulva, prepuce or anus can be used.

In addition to monitoring clinical signs, several items of monitoring equipment are recommended. Oesophageal stethoscopes allow direct assessment of cardiac rate and rhythm without disturbing the surgical field or draped area (Fig. 6.8). Systolic blood pressure should be measured wherever possible, and should be monitored if muscle relaxants are used. Normal blood pressure readings for dogs and cats, along with man for comparison, are listed in Table 6.5. Both oscillometric and Doppler flow methods are suitable, although the former provide information on diastolic as well as systolic blood pressure, along with mean arterial pressure and pulse rate (Fig. 6.9). Electrocardiogram recordings can detect changes in heart rhythm associated with cardiac pathology, or changes in electrolyte levels and hypoxia. Pulse oximetry is a non-invasive method for measuring arterial oxygen saturation. Positioning on the tongue may result in loss of readings as the surgeon moves his or her hands around the head. Placement on the vulva, teat or toe-web might be more reliable (Figs 6.6 and 6.10). Capnography measures exhaled carbon dioxide levels and gives an excellent measure of the adequacy of ventilation; its use is to be encouraged. Capnography should always be available if muscle relaxants are used. Both hypo- and hyperthermia can be encountered during anaes-

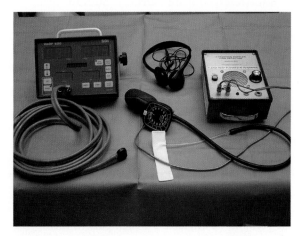

Fig. 6.9 Blood pressure monitors—oscillometric and Doppler.

Table 6.5 Normal blood pressure readings

Reading in mmHg	Dog	Cat	Man
Systolic `	110–190	120–170	110–140
Diastolic	55–110	70–120	70–100

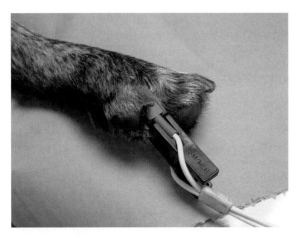

Fig. 6.10 Pulse oximeter placed on toe-web so as not to interfere with surgical access.

thesia and on recovery since the patient's ability to regulate body temperature is reduced.

Hypothermia is more common and delays recovery significantly—thus, frequent checks are advised. Core temperature (usually from the oesophagus with a thermistor or thermocouple, Fig. 6.8) is more reliable than rectal temperature, but the latter is better than no measurement at all! Fluids administered during surgery should also be checked, and any alterations in rates of infusion noted on the anaesthesia record sheet. Ideally, they should be warmed to reduce any hypothermic effect. Blood loss is usually minimal during ocular surgery, but might be significant with enucleations and should therefore be monitored.

Recovery

Provision for recovery should have been made when the anaesthetic plan was devised. A quiet, warm area should be available for each patient recovering from anaesthesia, and continued careful monitoring is required during this period. Soft comfortable bedding should be provided (e.g. Vet Bed), with incontinence pads since animals will frequently urinate or defecate on recovery. Body temperature should be measured frequently (hypothermia is a major cause of delayed recovery). Heat pads, reusable wheat-filled heat bags and bubble wrap or aluminium space blankets are useful.

Extubation of the ophthalmic patient should occur before the gag reflex is fully restored—but the patient must be sufficiently roused from unconsciousness to be able to protect the airway. This will prevent coughing and gagging which could lead to damage to the operated eye. However, care should be exercised with brachycephalics since the long soft palate can lead to obstruction, dyspnoea and respiratory distress if the tube is removed too early.

The patient should be positioned with the head extended and supported on bean bags if bilateral surgery has been performed. If surgery was unilateral, the operated eye should be uppermost (unless it has been a very long anaesthetic in which case the patient should be turned to reduce the risk of hypostatic congestion in the dependent, down-side lung). Pulse (rate and quality) and respiration should continue to be monitored along with temperature, mucous membrane colour and capillary refill time.

The wound can be gently cleaned with soft woven swabs moistened with sterile saline. This applies to procedures such as entropion surgery but not to intraocular surgery where skin incisions are rarely made (although occasionally a lateral canthotomy is performed). Topical medication might be necessary now. If an Elizabethan collar is to be used postoperatively, it can be fitted now, although it may cause some animals to panic and thrash about upon regaining consciousness, causing damage. It is often better to sit with the patient, gently talking to

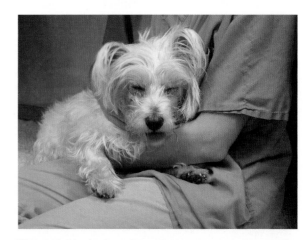

Fig. 6.11 Monitoring the patient on recovery from ocular surgery to prevent inadvertent damage to the eyes or wounds.

them as they wake (Fig. 6.11). This way they can be assessed for the presence of pain or irritation from the eye(s), as well as making sure that they do not bang or rub the eye(s). Foot bandages can be applied to prevent self-trauma. Care must be taken when moving patients back to their kennel, as they could bump into things due to a combination of disorientation following anaesthesia and impaired vision following the procedure. Intravenous catheters should only be removed when the animal has recovered fully from the effects of anaesthesia.

ANAESTHESIA IN PATIENTS WITH DIABETES MELLITUS

Special mention is made of diabetic patients since they commonly present for cataract evaluation and surgery. Ideally, the diabetes should be well-controlled before considering elective surgery. Any fluid deficits or ketoacidosis must be corrected prior to surgery. The normal medication routine is followed on the day prior to surgery. The owner should provide two or three meals for the patient and the current bottle of insulin in use. Try to disrupt the animal's regime as little as possible. Table 6.6 provides a checklist for diabetic patients.

Various protocols for anaesthesia of diabetic patients are available, but here we will outline only the most commonly followed regime. The surgery is planned for first thing in the morning, to enable careful monitoring on recovery and throughout the day. Food is not given in the morning, but water is freely available (diabetic patients are often polydipsic and can dehydrate very quickly). Blood glucose levels are measured and the patient is given half the normal morning dose of insulin at the time of premedication. The choice of premedication agent is important. Heavy sedatives must be avoided, as it is important that the patient wakes quickly and is able to eat once the surgery is finished. Only low doses of acepromazine should be used, combined with an opioid analgesic. Alpha-2-agonists should be avoided since they affect normal glucose homeostasis.

Fluid therapy is started and continued into the postoperative period. Various fluids can be used, such as 5% dextrose in water, 4.3% dextrose in 0.18% saline (which has the advantage over 5% dextrose in water, being a balanced solution that replaces fluid loss and provides sugar), Hartmann's or lactated Ringer's solution. The patient's blood glucose level is monitored every 30–45 minutes during surgery and on recovery (blood is collected from a separate site to which the fluid is administered). The placement of two catheters on premedication will ease sample collection. The aim is to keep glucose levels between 8–16 mmol/L during surgery. Altering the type of fluid administered, as well as the rate, will help to achieve this. Hypoglycaemia is more dangerous to the patient than short periods of hyperglycaemia.

Induction agents should be short-acting. Propofol is the preferred agent, although thiopental

Table 6.6 Checklist for diabetic patients undergoing hospitalisation and surgery	
Owner to provide the following	**Reason to be provided**
Current bottle of insulin	A slight difference in patient response might be noticed using a different or new bottle
Timetable of feeding and insulin injection, including amounts given	Aim to keep as close as possible to normal regime to reduce diabetic destabilisation
2 or 3 meals	Diabetics are often on special diets and the specific products might not be routinely stocked in the hospital
Any tips to encourage animal to eat if a picky eater, e.g. warming the food, stroking while feeding, feeding from a height	It is important that patients eat while hospitalised
Any concurrent eye or systemic medication	Continued medication will be required during hospitalisation

can also be used. For maintenance, isoflurane is better than halothane since it allows a rapid recovery. Any suitable breathing circuit can be used. Since muscle relaxants (neuromuscular-blocking agents) are usually used for cataract surgery, a suitable mechanical ventilator will also be used.

As soon as the animal is recovered from the anaesthetic, food is offered and if eaten the second half insulin dose is given. If the patient does not eat, no further insulin is given, but glucose levels are carefully monitored. The stress of hospitalisation, anaesthesia and surgery can upset diabetic stability, and blood glucose levels need to be frequently checked during the period of hospitalisation.

SEDATION FOR MINOR OPHTHALMIC PROCEDURES

Some ophthalmic procedures in dogs and cats can be performed under sedation with topical anaesthesia. Examples include sample and biopsy collection, nasolacrimal duct flushing, debridement and grid keratectomy for superficial corneal ulcers and electroretinography.

An alpha-2-adrenoceptor agonist such as medetomidine (Domitor, Pfizer) is commonly used for sedation and should be administered at moderate does rates (20–80 μ/kg). If more profound sedation is required, an opioid should be included (e.g. butorphanol, [Torbugesic, Fort Dodge]) which will increase the sedation without incurring further cardiopulmonary depression. A lower dose of meditomidine is used when combined with butorphanol. The latter is given at rates of 100–300 μg/kg in dogs and cats. Both agents can be combined in one syringe and given by subcutaneous, intramuscular or slow intravenous injection. The alpha-2-adrenoceptor agonist can be reversed with atipamazole (Antisedan, Pfizer) once the procedure is finished. It should be remembered that some animals are easily roused while under alpha-2-agonist sedation; they are often noise-sensitive, for example, and caution should be exercised. If sedated for a diagnostic procedure, such as nasolacrimal flushing for example, the eye could be damaged if the dog suddenly reacted to a door slamming or the telephone ringing.

Many other combinations of sedatives and analgesics, as well as dissociative anaesthetics such as ketamine (alone or in combination with other agents), can be employed to sedate patients for minor procedures. Reference to specific texts should be made for the advantages and disadvantages of these. Surgeon preference and familiarity with the agents available will influence the choice of sedative.

RABBIT ANAESTHESIA

Rabbits frequently suffer from ocular problems, which sometimes require surgical intervention. They are not generally fasted prior to surgery (they have a very tight gastric sphincter which prevents vomiting, and starving can induce detrimental ileus). Neuroleptanalgesic drugs (fentanyl–fluanisone combination [Hypnorm, Janssen]) can be used as a premedicant, sedative or part of an injectable anaesthetic. It is usually given intramuscularly 20 minutes before induction. Induction can follow with intravenous (via ear vein) diazepam or midazolam, and this combination provides good analgesia, muscle relaxation and about 20–30 minutes of anaesthesia. Dose rates for all agents used in rabbits can be found in the relevant data sheets or specialised texts.

Alternatively, induction can be achieved with ketamine and medetomidine, or ketamine and xylazine. Masking down is not recommended for ocular procedures and can induce severe hypoxia following breath holding, in addition to the potential ocular trauma through struggling. After induction using an injectable agent, anaesthesia can be maintained with inhalational agents. Isoflurane is preferred to halothane. Intubation is more difficult in rabbits than dogs and cats but can be achieved with the help of a paediatric laryngoscope and a specialised rabbit gag. Lignocaine spray directed onto the larynx and the use of guide-wires can also assist intubation. Complications with rabbit anaesthesia include respiratory depression and hypoxia, along with cardiac arrhythmias and even cardiac arrest. Intermittent positive pressure ventilation can help (via a tight-fitting face mask if no endotracheal tube is placed). Rabbits are normally positioned in lateral recumbency for eye surgery. They should be placed on heated pads and wrapped in aluminium space blankets or bubble wrap to minimise heat loss and hypothermia. Monitoring should be adapted, bearing in mind the different responses in rabbits (e.g. retention of a pedal withdrawal reflex even in relatively deep planes of anaesthesia). Close monitoring is required throughout the recovery period. Customised Elizabethan collars (e.g. those designed for birds) can be used to prevent rubbing the eyes.

EQUINE ANAESTHESIA

The same principles of anaesthesia that apply to small animals also apply to horses. However, the sheer size of equine patients creates some difficulties and can increase the risk of injury to staff as well as the animal. A detailed discussion of equine anaesthesia is beyond the scope of this book, but we can mention some relevant points here.

For simple ocular surgery, such as repairing eyelid lacerations, removing superficial foreign bodies and taking biopsy samples, sedation and either topical anaesthesia or regional nerve blocks are used in the standing horse. Sedation is typically achieved by using an alpha-2-adrenoceptor agent (e.g. xylazine or detomidine), often combined with an opioid such as butorphanol. Additional anaesthesia can be achieved using nerve blocks.

The auriculopalpebral nerve (branch of the facial nerve [cranial nerve VII]) is most commonly blocked, which prevents blinking but not sensation (Fig. 6.12). It must be combined with topical anaesthesia to block corneal sensitivity, or a supraorbital nerve (branch of trigeminal, cranial

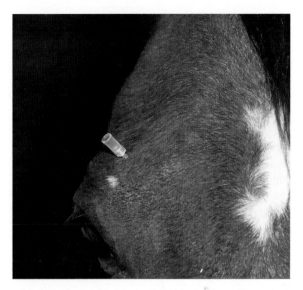

Fig. 6.13 Supraorbital nerve block in a horse. (Photograph courtesy of Dr. Dennis Brooks, University of Florida)

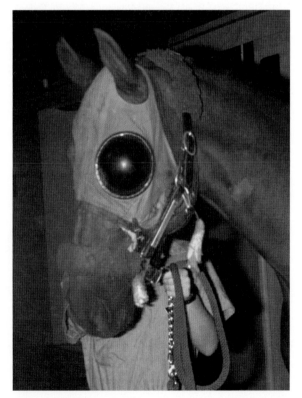

Fig. 6.14 Head collar with eye cup to prevent ocular damage. (Photograph courtesy of Dr. Dennis Brooks, University of Florida)

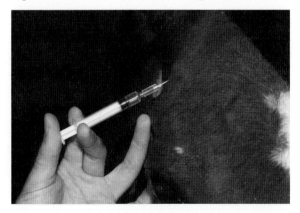

Fig. 6.12 Auriculopalpebral nerve block in a horse. (Photograph courtesy of Dr. Dennis Brooks, University of Florida)

nerve V) block to desensitise the medial $^2/_3$ of the upper lid (Fig. 6.13). If general anaesthesia is required it should be undertaken in an equine hospital and not 'in the field'.

General anaesthesia in horses follows the same stages as in small animals. Premedication is often achieved with an alpha-2-adrenoceptor agonist, such as xylazine and detomidine. Further analgesia can be achieved with NSAIDs. General anaesthesia can be induced with intravenous (via a jugular catheter) ketamine or thiopental; endotracheal intubation is performed and either halothane or isoflurane in oxygen can be used to maintain anaesthesia via a rebreathing circuit (e.g. circle). Monitoring is similar to small animals, although continuous ECG monitoring and direct arterial pressure measurements are highly recommended.

Recovery from general anaesthesia is a critical time for horses. A quiet, dimly lit (ideally via a dimmer switch), padded room is advised for anaesthetic recovery and the patient must be closely observed while it tries to get up and remains ataxic, since damage to the eye could occur if the animal bangs its head. The lateral placement of equine eyes makes them particularly vulnerable, and a protective head collar with eye cup might be advised as shown in Figure 6.14.

BIBLIOGRAPHY AND FURTHER READING

Bishop Y. The veterinary formulary. 6th edn. London: Pharmaceutical press; 2004

Coumbe KM, ed. Equine veterinary nursing manual. Oxford: Blackwell Science; 2001.

Lane DR, Cooper B, eds. Veterinary nursing. 3rd edn. Oxford: Butterworth Heinemann; 2003.

Moore AH, ed. BSAVA manual of advanced veterinary nursing. Gloucester: British Small Animal Veterinary Association; 1999.

Moore M, ed. BSAVA Manual of veterinary nursing. Gloucester: British Small Animal Veterinary Association; 1999.

Welsh E, ed. Anaesthesia for veterinary nurses. Oxford: Blackwell Science; 2003.

7 General ophthalmic conditions

INTRODUCTION

In this chapter we review some common ophthalmic conditions, mainly in dogs and cats, but a section is included on rabbits and other small mammals and exotics at the end of the chapter.

We will be discussing conditions which are seen in general and ophthalmology practice, including their management (more advanced and specialised treatments are discussed in Chapter 8). This chapter does not provide an exhaustive list of all eye problems encountered—for this you need to refer to an ophthalmology textbook. However, I have included the most commonly encountered conditions which as a nurse you will be directly involved with. Each condition is highlighted as requiring either primarily medical M or surgical treatment S, although for some diseases a combination of both will be necessary M S (e.g. glaucoma or progressing corneal ulcers). If neither symbol is present either no treatment is available, or none is required. A summary of the nursing requirements is shown in Table 7.1 (for more specific details refer to Chapters 4 and 5). We will start at the front of the eye and work our way through to the back.

SUMMARY OF SYMBOLS

M —mainly medical nursing

S —mainly surgical nursing

M S —combination nursing often required

No symbol—No treatment possible or none required

Table 7.1 General nursing care for ophthalmic patients

Medical
- Clean and bathe eye as required
- Draw up a timetable for medication
- Apply topical and systemic medication as prescribed
- Prevent self trauma
- Attend to general nursing of the patient
- Fill out discharge sheet for owner
- Show owner how to apply medication
- Explain to owner what to expect regarding progress
- Make recheck appointment for owner

Surgical
- Prepare patient for surgery
- Prepare theatre and necessary equipment
- Get all instrument kits and suture material ready
- Check with surgeon whether any extra items are required
- Assist during procedure as required
- Recover patient from surgery
- Apply any immediate postoperative medication required
- Liaise with hospital nurse regarding post operative care

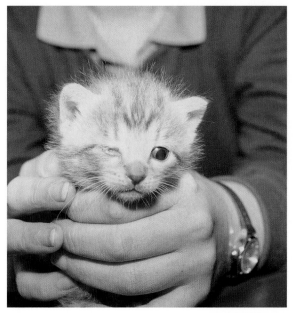

Fig. 7.1 Ophthalmia neonatorum affecting the right eye of this kitten.

ADNEXA

The adnexa is the term given to the accessory ocular structures, i.e. the eyelids, conjunctiva and nasolacrimal system. The orbit and its contents can also be included in the definition, although this is discussed separately below. Conditions affecting the adnexal structures are very common in veterinary ophthalmology.

Eyelids

Congenital problems

Ophthalmia neonatorum M

The eyelids of dogs and cats are normally closed at birth. A pin-point opening develops at the medial canthus, which then gradually enlarges and the eyes open by 10–14 days. The eye is not fully developed at birth, and this continued lid closure protects the immature cornea and conjunctiva. Occasionally, lid opening fails to occur and the risk of infection beneath the closed lids becomes quite high. Ophthalmia neonatorum (neonatal conjunctivitis) is the name given to infections within the conjunctiva behind the closed lids (Fig. 7.1). Staphylococcal infections are most common, and organisms might contaminate the eyes during birth (from the dam's genital tract). Often more than one member of the litter is affected, and the condition can affect one or both eyes.

Treatment entails opening the eyelids: one blade from a pair of small blunt-ended scissors is inserted at the medial canthus parallel to the lids, and the palpebral fissure is gently opened. Samples of the discharge are taken for culture and sensitivity.

Nursing care is critical for these neonatal patients. Specific care will include frequent bathing of the discharge. Cotton buds moistened with sterile saline can be used, with a separate bud for each eye. Once the discharge is removed, a broad-spectrum antibiotic ointment is applied at least 4× daily while awaiting the culture and sensitivity results. The corneal surface must be kept moist, particularly if the lids have been opened early to release the infection, since normal blinking and tear production will not yet have been developed. Ocular lubricants might be required in addition to the antibiotics. Most infections respond well to this approach, but corneal ulceration and even rupture can occur in a few cases. Blindness or even loss of the eye can result. In addition to specific treatment for the eyes, general nursing of the neonate will be required; for example, they might require supplementary feeding and cleaning.

Eyelid agenesis (coloboma) S

A coloboma is an absence of tissue and is occasionally seen in puppies but more commonly in kittens. It is usually the outer portion of the upper lid that is missing, such that proper blinking cannot take place and fur from the surrounding skin rubs directly on the cornea. This causes irritation and ulceration. Surgical reconstruction is required. Small defects can be repaired by a simple realignment of the remaining lid margins, but large defects require sliding skin flaps. Often more than two procedures are required before an acceptable result is obtained.

Dermoid S

A dermoid is a piece of normal skin located in an abnormal position. Dermoids can occur anywhere in the body, but around the eye they are most common on the conjunctiva and cornea, and sometimes affecting the lids. They grow as the animal does, and usually need to be surgically removed as the abnormal hairs rub on the cornea and cause ulceration. If a significant portion of the cornea is affected, referral for a surgical keratectomy using an operating microscope is advised.

Acquired conditions of the eyelids

Acquired conditions of the lids are numerous. They can include entropion, ectropion, eyelash problems, injuries, inflammation of the lids (blepharitis), neoplasia and conditions affecting the third eyelid.

Entropion S

Entropion is an in-rolling of the eyelid and is a common, developmental, often breed-related problem (Fig. 7.2). Young pedigree dogs, such as the Labrador retriever, chow chow and rottweiler,

present at a few months of age (Fig. 7.3). Shar-pei puppies can be affected at only a few weeks of age (Fig. 7.4). Typical signs are blepharospasm (increased blinking), increased lacrimation and corneal ulceration affecting one or both eyes.

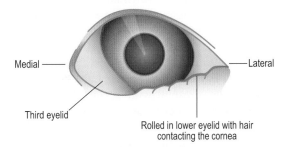

Fig. 7.2 Entropion of the lower eyelid affecting the lateral $^2/_3$. (From Grahn 2004, with permission of Butterworth Heinemann)

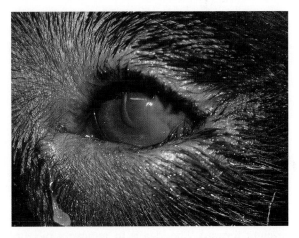

Fig. 7.3 Rottweiler with entropion causing marked corneal ulceration and vascularisation.

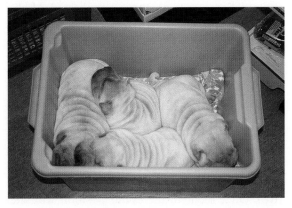

Fig. 7.4 Litter of Shar-pei puppies all with entropion.

Surgery should not be delayed until the animal reaches maturity, as used to be recommended; this only prolongs the discomfort to the animal and can lead to permanent corneal damage. Anaesthetic agents are now much safer, and surgery can be safely performed in young animals. If necessary, a second procedure can be undertaken later in life if the entropion returns as the animal grows. The entropion affects different parts of the eyelids, depending on the breed conformation. For example, young Labrador retrievers typically present with a lateral lower lid entropion, while Persian cats are seen with a lower lid medial entropion. Shar-pei dogs often have severe in-rolling of all four eyelids!

Other types of entropion include spastic entropion which develops secondary to a painful eye, such as with a corneal ulcer. Ongoing blepharospasm allows the lid to roll inwards, and this rubs on the cornea causing more discomfort and the onset of a vicious cycle. Treating the initiating problem (e.g. the corneal ulcer) will sometimes correct the entropion, but spasm of the lid muscles can be permanent such that some animals do require corrective surgery.

Senile entropion is most common in older cocker spaniels. They lose skin elasticity and everything starts to sag (so called 'slipped facial mask' with the dog presenting with a sad-looking expression as shown in Fig. 7.5). This causes the upper eyelids to roll in and rub on the cornea.

In most cases, surgery for entropion is quite straight forward. The idea is to remove a piece of skin from close to the eyelid margin which will result in the lid sitting flat against the eye when sutured. Some cases are more complicated. Medial entropion is best corrected with the assistance of magnification (ideally an operating microscope). Some entropion is associated with laxity of the ligament at the lateral canthus, which also needs to be addressed, while some patients have very poor anatomy with a combination if entropion and ectropion (diamond eye). Complicated surgery is discussed in Chapter 8.

For all entropion surgery, it is important that the patient is fully assessed by the surgeon prior to the administration of any premedication or sedatives. Once sedated, the eyelid position will alter making it very difficult to assess exactly how much

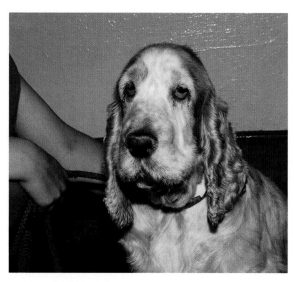

Fig. 7.5 Elderly cocker spaniel with slipped facial mask resulting in entropion of the upper eyelids.

tissue needs to be removed. Thus, the nurse should always check with the surgeon before giving any premedication. The sutures used around the eye need to be soft and non-irritating. Often absorbable material is chosen to avoid the need for suture removal which could necessitate sedation, with the sutures being so close to the eye.

Nursing after the surgery will entail making sure that the patient does not attempt to rub. This often happens during the recovery from anaesthesia, and simply sitting with the patient to prevent this is often all that is needed. Once fully awake, it is likely that the patient will be much more comfortable than prior to the operation since the eyelids are no longer rubbing on the cornea. Elizabethan collars are not usually required (although some dogs will insist on trying to undo the surgeon's work!). Topical antibiotics are usually prescribed, especially if ulceration is present, but in some cases dogs are discharged with only systemic therapy. This is to prevent drawing attention to the eyes with the frequent application of medication. Many dogs, especially breeds like rottweilers and great Danes, will become head shy and as soon as anyone approaches the face will start to squint and encourage further blepharospasm, leading to more entropion (the vicious cycle mentioned above).

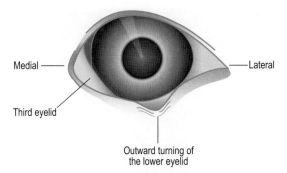

Medial

Lateral

Third eyelid

Outward turning of
the lower eyelid

Fig. 7.6 Ectropion of the lower eyelid. (From Grahn 2004, with permission of Butterworth Heinemann)

Thus, minimal handling and systemic NSAIDs are usually sufficient treatment.

Ectropion S

Ectropion is the rolling out of the eyelids (Fig. 7.6) and is less irritating than entropion. It most commonly affects the lower lids and is associated with the lids being too long. It is often worse when the animal is tired. The conjunctiva becomes inflamed through exposure, and mucus and debris build-up in the lower conjunctival sac, leading to conjunctivitis and secondary infection. Breeds most commonly affected include cocker spaniels, basset hounds, bloodhounds and Saint Bernards. In addition, ectropion can result from over-correction of entropion. The most simple way to correct the condition is to shorten the lid by removing a full-thickness wedge of tissue. However, dogs with diamond eye will require shortening of the lid, entropion surgery for the parts which roll inwards and usually stabilisation of the lateral canthus. This surgery is complicated! Many different procedures have been described and can be adapted to the individual needs of the patient. Post-operative nursing is similar to that for entropion, as described above.

Eyelash abnormalities S

Eyelash abnormalities are more common in dogs than cats. Several different conditions are seen, depending on the exact location of the lashes, and include trichiasis, distichiasis and ectopic cilia (see Table 7.2 for definitions).

Trichiasis is normal facial hair rubbing on the ocular surface. Normal eyelashes, fur from a prominent nasal fold or hair on the caruncle (the small fleshy protuberance at the medial canthus) can all cause problems. The most common form of trichiasis is probably that seen in older cocker spaniels with facial droop. In such cases a true entropion can be present, although often there is just irritation from the hairs along the upper lid rubbing on the eye. Surgical correction can include procedures just at the eyelid margin, or a total 'face-lift' in more severe cases. Chronic conjunctivitis and keratitis are usually present along with the eyelash problem, and medical management for these is also required.

If nasal folds are in contact with the cornea (e.g. in Pekinese and pugs), surgical resection is required. For caruncle hairs causing a clinical problem, either resection of the offending tissue or cryosurgery can be employed.

Distichiasis is the presence of extra eyelashes along the eyelid margin (Fig. 7.7), although in many cases the lashes do not actually cause any problem. Breeds most commonly affected include cocker spaniels (both American and English varieties), miniature long-haired dachshunds, Staffordshire bull terriers, English bulldogs, boxers and weimaraners. Cats only occasionally suffer from distichiasis. If the extra lashes are soft and floating in the tear film, they are unlikely to be irritating to the dog. However, blepharospasm, increased lacrimation and rubbing of the eyes will suggest that the irritation is significant. Young dogs are most likely to have problems.

Table 7.2 Definitions of eyelash abnormalities

Name	Description
Trichiasis	Hair in a normal position rubbing on the eyeball, e.g. from nasal folds or eyelids
Distichiasis	Extra row of lashes along the eyelid margin
Ectopic cilia (singular, cilium)	Lashes growing through the eyelid conjunctiva, rubbing on the cornea

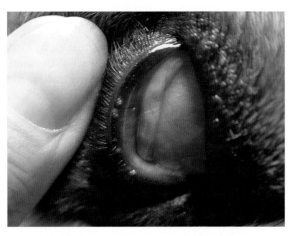

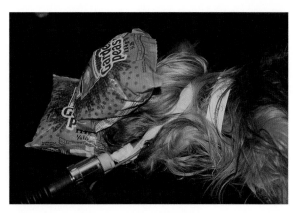

Fig. 7.8 Ice packs (in this case bags of frozen peas which mould well against the eyelids!) placed to reduce swelling following cryosurgery for distichiasis.

Fig. 7.7 Distichiasis (cilia on the eyelid margin, several visible) plus ectopic cilium in the palpebral conjunctiva.

Simply plucking the lashes will temporarily relive the clinical signs but as soon as the cilia regrow, the problems will return. More permanent methods of lash removal include electrolysis and cryosurgery. Electrolysis should be performed under good magnification since the epilation needle needs to be inserted accurately alongside each lash. If the needle is misplaced the hair follicle will not be destroyed and the lash will grow back. Electrolysis can be very time consuming if multiple lashes are present. Cryosurgery is less refined. The eyelid adjacent to the lashes is frozen with the probe, and this damages the hair follicle so that no regrowth should occur. However, the eyelids swell dramatically after cryosurgery and the owners must be warned. Ice packs should be available and applied immediately after the procedure (Fig. 7.8). Systemic NSAIDs as well as topical antibiotic/ steroid combinations are used for a couple of weeks after the surgery. The eyelid margin can depigment following cryosurgery; it usually is only temporary but can cause concern to some owners. Client education by the nurse prior to the procedure is advised. Occasionally, distichia can be surgically resected by removing the hair follicles through the palpebral eyelid margin. However, these procedures can easily lead to lid scarring (which can be more severe than the distichiasis), so are not recommended unless the surgeon has had special training.

Ectopic cilia are lashes which grow through the palpebral conjunctiva to rub directly on the corneal surface (Fig. 7.7). These are always clinically relevant, and ulceration is common. Single lashes are most frequent but small groups do occasionally grow. Flat coated retrievers commonly present with ectopic cilia, but they can be seen in any breed, especially those which also suffer from distichiasis. Typically, a young dog presents with unilateral blepharospasm and an ulcer in the dorsal part of the cornea. It is important to evert the upper lid to look for a lash—without magnification they can be very difficult to see. If distichia are also present these may be blamed for the discomfort, but with an ectopic cilium the pain and ulceration are usually much worse. Once identified, it is fairly simple surgery to remove the lash. The offending hair is excised along with the follicle under general anaesthesia with magnification. A chalazion clamp to stabilise the lid and provide haemostasis makes the procedure more straight forward (Fig. 5.14, p. 71). Suturing is not necessary. Nursing afterwards is minimal since the dog is likely to be much more comfortable. If ulceration is present, topical antibiotics should be used until the cornea has healed.

Eyelid injuries S

Injuries to the eyelids are quite common in dogs and cats. Bite wounds, scratches and road traffic accidents can all lead to damage. Initial first aid treatment should comprise of cold compresses (a flannel or soft cloth wrapped around crushed ice cubes is ideal) to provide haemostasis and minimise swelling. The patient should be fully examined to check for other injuries. In general, it is best to repair eyelid lacerations early—unless grossly infected when wound reconstruction is delayed until the infection has been controlled. The eyelids are very vascular and tend to heal quickly. Close attention to accurate lid margin alignment is vital to retain proper blink function and tear film distribution. Poor surgery can result in scarring, entropion, ectropion or trichiasis. If the injury is located medially, it is important that nasolacrimal function is checked—lacerations involving the punctae require specialist microsurgical repair.

Eyelid inflammation (blepharitis) M   S

Inflammation of the eyelids is frequently encountered in dogs (less so in cats). It can be localised to one area of the lid, affect all of both lids, or be associated with more widespread dermatitis. Blepharitis can result from:

- allergic causes such as atopy or contact sensitivity
- bacterial infections
- immune-mediated responses
- parasitic infections (e.g. sarcoptic or demodectic mange)
- self-inflicted inflammation due to rubbing for another ocular problem.

Obviously, identifying the underlying cause by a thorough ocular and clinical examination with the use of skin scrapes, swabs for bacterial culture and biopsy if necessary will allow for appropriate treatment.

Abscesses of the lid margin (normally of the meibomian glands) result in a painful eye (hordeolum) or non-painful chalazium (plural, chalazia). Both appear as nodular yellowish masses along the conjunctival surface of the lids. Drainage and the use of warm compresses will result in a quicker resolution than the use of antibiotics alone.

Meibomianitis manifests as swollen inflamed eyelids which on close inspection have multiple cream-coloured swellings along the conjunctiva close to the lid margin. If gently squeezed, discharge is released along the lid margin through the meibomian openings. This should be cultured.

The condition can follow a bacterial conjunctivitis (e.g. with staphylococcal agents). Medical management involves topical and systemic antibiotics, and sometimes anti-inflammatory agents. Good nursing with regular bathing and warm compresses will assist.

Immune-mediated blepharitis rarely occurs alone—other clinical signs are usually present (e.g. at other mucocutaneous junctions). Biopsy and histopathology will confirm the diagnosis such that appropriate medical management can be instigated.

Eyelid neoplasia S

Tumours of the eyelids occur in both dogs and cats—usually older patients. Many canine tumours are benign, and most commonly include sebaceous adenomas, papillomas and melanomas. However, squamous cell carcinomas are quite common in cats, and these are more aggressive with local invasion and spread to regional lymph nodes. Cytology should be performed on suspicious lesions. In general, early excision and histopathological examination is recommended. Small lesions are more easily removed without the need for extensive reconstructive surgery. Some tumours are sensitive to cryosurgery, which can be performed under sedation and local anaesthesia in cooperative patients.

Conditions of the nictitating membrane (third eyelid)

The nictitating membrane is found ventromedially between the eyelids and globe. It provides protection, helps to spread the tears evenly across the corneal surface and removes debris. It can be involved in several pathological processes—most commonly injuries, prolapse of the nictitans gland, scrolled cartilage and inflammatory conditions. The 'third eyelid flap' is a commonly performed surgical procedure in general practice.

Injuries to the third eyelid S

The nictitans membrane is quite commonly damaged during cat fights and occasionally as dogs run through bramble bushes or similar. Since it is well vascularised, the nictitans membrane tends to bleed readily so immediate nursing attention should include applying gentle pressure to the area with a moistened gauze swab, taking care not to put direct pressure on the eye itself since this could also be injured. Once a thorough ophthalmic examination has been undertaken and the extent of damage ascertained, a treatment plan can be formulated. It is essential to check that no foreign body is retained—pieces of cat claw can get trapped in the membrane or in the conjunctival fornix. Fluorescein should be used to assess whether any corneal damage is present, but hopefully the third eyelid will have done its job in protecting the cornea. Tears in the nictitans membrane should be surgically repaired wherever possible. Careful attention to the leading edge of the third eyelid should be paid—the correct anatomical alignment of this area is essential to maintain proper function. Sometimes, small tears parallel to the free edge of the membrane will leave flaps of free tissue which need to be trimmed off. Nursing post-surgery will entail preventing self trauma and usually the use of broad-spectrum antibiotics.

Prolapse of the nictitans gland (cherry eye) S

Prolapse of the gland of the third eyelid is very common in certain breeds of dogs, including English bulldogs, great Danes, dogues de Bordeaux, Neopolitan and other mastiff breeds (Fig. 7.9). It is occasionally seen in cats, particularly Burmese.

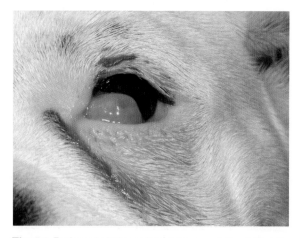

Fig. 7.9 Prolapsed nictitans gland (cherry eye) in a 4-month-old bulldog.

The gland is normally located deep within the membrane of the third eyelid, but pops out of position and is seen as a smooth pink mass protruding from behind the membrane. Both eyes are usually affected, but not always simultaneously. The gland produces about $1/3$ of the aqueous portion of tears and should not be removed. Many of the breeds susceptible to cherry eye are also predisposed to keratoconjunctivitis sicca, and this can be exacerbated if the gland has been excised. Thus, surgical repositioning is recommended. There are several techniques for doing this, and surgeon preference together with the breed will influence the choice of method. Owners should be warned that the nictitans membrane will remain swollen and inflamed for up to a couple of weeks after the surgery. Postoperative nursing care will usually entail topical ointments—antibiotics or antibiotic/anti-inflammatory combinations depending on the degree of glandular swelling.

Scrolling of the third eyelid S

The third eyelid has a piece of cartilage within its substance which helps to maintain its shape. Unfortunately, in some breeds the cartilage is weak and kinks over, resulting in a bend in its centre. This deforms the membrane and reduces its functional capacity. It can be seen in conjunction with prolapse of the nictitans gland or in isolation. Breeds affected include those listed for cherry eye, as well as weimaraners and other large sporting breeds. The weakened piece of cartilage needs to be surgically resected to allow the third eyelid to sit flat against the corneal surface again. Sutures are not normally required and nursing aftercare is minimal—usually just topical antibiotics for a few days to prevent infection.

Inflammatory conditions affecting the third eyelid M

Inflammatory conditions of the nictitans membrane are seen occasionally. Sometimes owners think that the third eyelid is inflamed if it lacks pigment at the leading edge. This is just a normal variation, but when seen unilaterally (e.g. in spaniel breeds) the membrane will be more obvious on the non-pigmented side since the pink colour contrasts with the iris colour, whereas on the pigmented side it tends to blend in more. Once the colour difference has been pointed out no action is required!

Plasma cell infiltration of the third eyelids (plasmoma) is seen in German and Belgian shepherd dogs and their crossbreeds, and sometimes in greyhounds and lurchers. The membranes are thickened with a cobble-stone appearance and become bright pink in colour. The condition is considered immune-mediated and usually responds to topical medication with cilcosporin or steroids. Life-long medication is normally necessary to prevent relapses. It can be seen alone or in conjunction with chronic superficial keratitis (pannus), which is discussed later (p. 118).

The third eyelid will also be inflamed with many generalised ophthalmic conditions (e.g. conjunctivitis, blepharitis, uveitis, etc.), and a thorough ocular examination is necessary to check whether other ocular structures are involved.

Neoplasia of the third eyelid M S

Neoplasia of the third eyelid is rare, but many tumour types can be encountered, such as squamous cell carcinoma, lymphoma and adenocarcinoma. Biopsy and histological determination of tissue type are necessary before deciding on a treatment plan. Confirmed neoplasia is the only indication for total excision of the membrane.

Third eyelid flap S

The third eyelid flap is a common surgical procedure in general practice, although it is rarely used by veterinary ophthalmologists. The procedure is used mainly for non-infected superficial corneal ulcers to provide some limited protection and promote comfort during healing. However, the cornea cannot be examined while the flap is in situ, and as such it is possible for the ulcer to be getting worse without the owners or veterinary surgeon being aware of this. In the procedure, the third eyelid is drawn across the cornea under general anaesthesia and can be sutured either to the bulbar conjunctiva or to the upper lid. The first technique is preferred since the third eyelid then moves with the eyeball, and more protection is offered. If the third eyelid is sutured to the

upper lid, the eye moves independently beneath and the damaged cornea can still rub against the bulbar side of the third eyelid, slowing healing. However, suturing to the upper lid has the supposed advantage of allowing the suture knots to be undone, the cornea checked, and the suture retied without needing to operate again.

When the sutures are placed in the third eyelid it is important that they do not penetrate the cartilage but go around it instead. They should not perforate the full thickness of the third eyelid since this would result in rubbing on the cornea, exacerbating the ulceration! Suture material must be soft and non-irritating—silk or polygalatin 910 (Vicryl, Ethicon) are commonly employed. The flap is left in place for 7–10 days before being taken down to assess healing. It can be replaced if necessary, but if successful healing has not taken place after 2–3 weeks, other methods of treatment should be considered.

Conjunctiva M

Conditions of the conjunctiva are very commonly encountered. Conjunctivitis is inflammation of the conjunctiva and can occur as a condition in its own right or along with other, potentially more serious ocular conditions. It can be seen in animals of any age and can be primary (e.g. infectious) or secondary (e.g. associated with mechanical damage from entropion). Clinical signs include hyperaemia, chemosis and increased ocular discharge and are detailed in Table 7.3. The discharge can range from serous lacrimation to overt purulent material. Conjunctivitis tends to be irritating rather than overtly painful. Infectious agents include primary viruses such as distemper in dogs and feline herpes virus (see below), secondary bacterial infections (often streptococci or staphylococci) and *Chlamydophila* in cats (which can be primary or secondary). Irritants, such as wind, dust, chemicals or sometimes topically applied drugs, can cause conjunctivitis. Allergies also commonly cause conjunctivitis—usually bilaterally and more frequently in dogs than cats.

The diagnosis of conjunctivitis will include a full ophthalmic and clinical examination, including Schirmer tear test readings, cytology samples

Table 7.3 Ophthalmic signs of conjunctivitis

Clinical sign	Appearance
Conjunctival hyperaemia	Redness of ocular surface
Chemosis	Swelling of conjunctiva
Increased lacrimation	Tear overflow
Mucopurulent discharge	Yellow or green sticky discharge
Follicle formation in chronic cases	Cobblestone appearance to conjunctiva
Irritation and self trauma	Periorbital redness and hair loss

and swabs for bacterial culture and sensitivity testing. Conjunctival biopsy samples will sometimes be taken. Once the underlying cause is established, specific treatment can be prescribed. In addition to bathing any discharge regularly, topical medication such as antibiotics or anti-inflammatories will be used.

Traumatic conjunctivitis, such as due to blunt trauma, will result in subconjunctival haemorrhage. This can look dramatic but is usually not too severe, providing intraocular contents are undamaged. Symptomatic treatment is all that is required.

Systemic illnesses can also affect the conjunctiva (e.g. anaemia produces pallid conjunctival surfaces; jaundice, yellowed; cyanosis, mauve). Thus, the colour of the conjunctiva is very important and should always be monitored in hospitalised patients, especially those in intensive care. Small haemorrhages might indicate an underlying clotting problem. If noted, a complete clinical examination is warranted to look for systemic disease. Ocular manifestations of systemic disease are outlined later in this chapter (p. 139).

Cat 'flu' M

The agents which target the feline respiratory tract (feline herpes virus [FHV-1], calicivirus and *Chlamydophila*) can all be involved with cat flu, and ocular signs are very common. Feline upper respiratory tract disease (FLURD) refers to FHV-1 and calicivirus. The degree of involvement of the respiratory system and eyes will depend on which agent is present, and mixed infections are quite common. The syndrome is more common and severe in multi-cat households. Incubation periods are a matter of days (2–10 days usually) and all agents involved are highly contagious. Transmission is via direct contact with ocular or nasal discharges, and sneezing will cause spread via aerosols. Prevention is via vaccination. Secondary bacterial infections often accompany the disease.

Neonatal infections tend to be more severe than those in older kittens and adults. Ophthalmia neonatorum was mentioned in the section on congenital eyelid problems (p.104), and when associated with FHV-1 the severe conjunctivitis can progress to corneal ulceration and even perforation, as well as panophthalmitis and loss of the eye. If the eyelids are still fused, they should be gently opened with delicate blunt-tipped scissors. In slightly older kittens, an acute bilateral conjunctivitis with accompanying respiratory signs is the most common presentation. Chemosis is severe, and corneal ulceration can occur (Fig. 7.10). A serous ocular discharge soon becomes mucopurulent, with secondary bacterial contamination. The discharge is often thick and profuse, such that the eyelids become stuck together.

Nursing care is vital for these kittens. Barrier nursing to prevent cross infection must be maintained. Specific ophthalmic nursing will include frequent removal of ocular discharges by gentle bathing, application of broad-spectrum antibiotic agents topically, along with ocular lubricants and sometimes topical antiviral drops. General nursing support will be required—cleansing nasal discharges, supplementary feeding and intravenous fluids in severe cases. Systemic antibiotics are usually necessary, along with decongestants in some cats.

Infections in adult cats tend to cause only mild respiratory signs, along with conjunctivitis or keratitis with FHV-1. Many cats which recover from the initial infection remain carriers and can shed the virus from time to time. They will show mild

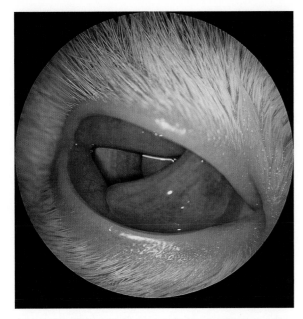

Fig. 7.10 Severe conjunctivitis and chemosis in a 5-month-old cat with FHV-1. Both eyes were affected, ulcers developed and upper respiratory signs were also present.

symptoms intermittently throughout life, particularly when stressed or ill. Other complications of cat flu include symblepharon (adhesions of conjunctiva to itself or to the cornea), blocked nasolacrimal ducts, keratoconjunctivitis sicca, sequestrum formation (p. 117) and recurrent ulceration.

Nasolacrimal system

Conditions which affect the nasolacrimal system can be broadly divided into those affecting the secretory component and those affecting drainage. Problems in the secretory elements can be further subdivided into excessive production (increased lacrimation) and reduced production (keratoconjunctivitis sicca). Tears are produced by the lacrimal and accessory glands, and are composed of an aqueous layer (the majority) together with mucous and oily layers (p. 4). Drainage is via the nasolacrimal punctae and nasolacrimal duct to the nose and the back of the mouth. Investigations of nasolacrimal system dysfunction include:

- evaluation of tear production using Schirmer tear tests

- assessment of conformation (including size and position) of the nasolacrimal punctae
- checking for the presence of hairs around the eyes
- assessment of the nature of any discharge.

Nasolacrimal cannulation and flushing might also be necessary, as might sample collection for laboratory investigation, fluorescein staining and contrast radiography in some cases. These procedures are all discussed in Chapter 3.

Tear overflow/ocular discharge M S

Over production of tears (excessive lacrimation) is usually due to a painful condition, such as a corneal ulcer. Schirmer tear test readings will be excessive, and the eye will appear wet and will be inflamed. The cause for the increased lacrimation should be obvious on clinical examination, and once this is treated (e.g. surgery for entropion , or the removal of an ectopic cilium), the lacrimation should reduce to normal levels.

Tear overflow or epiphora can result from developmental abnormalities, such as the absence of nasolacrimal punctae (imperforate punctae) or the presence of very small openings (micropunctae). These can be surgically enlarged or created, and will restore proper drainage. Magnification with an operating microscope renders the surgery straight forward.

Miniature breeds, such as toy poodles and Shi Tzus, commonly suffer from epiphora (Fig. 7.11a). Tear staining is obvious, particularly in white animals or those with white faces (e.g. bichon frise). Usually the owners are far more concerned than the dog, as no irritation or pain is associated with the condition. It occurs due to a number of contributing factors: a shallow orbit and prominent globe, close apposition of the eyelids, medial lower lid entropion functionally closing over the ventral nasolacrimal punctum, medial canthal hairs, distichiasis, hairs on the caruncles and misplacement of the nasolacrimal punctae. It can be challenging to establish which of these features is most relevant in some dogs since many have several abnormalities! Normally cannulation of the nasolacrimal system and flushing is easily performed, although fluorescein dye fails to exit from the nose but instead flows over the face after application to

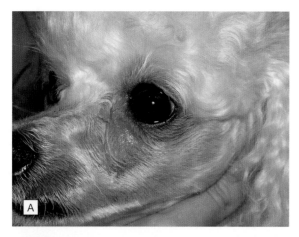

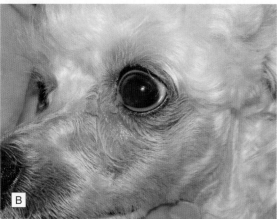

Fig. 7.11 Epiphora: a) poodle with epiphora; b) fluorescein flows over the face.

the eye (adding to the discolouration!)(Fig. 7.11b). This shows that although the nasolacrimal system is anatomically patent, functionally it is not! True anatomical abnormalities can be corrected with surgery (entropion surgery or removing hairs from the caruncles) but often just frequently wiping away the tears will suffice. Owners should be dissuaded from using astringent washes to try to remove the discolouration—these will sting if splashed into the eyes and can lead to sore skin and a moist dermatitis.

Epiphora can be an acquired condition—inflammation of the nasolacrimal system can result in stenosis of the duct, leading to permanent tear overflow. Feline herpes virus can cause similar blockages affecting either the duct and/or punctae. Foreign bodies and masses pressing on the duct will also lead to overflow. Nasolacrimal flush-ing and cannulation of the ducts with fine nylon to help locate a blockage will be necessary. Contrast radiography is sometimes employed to assist the diagnosis. Some cases can be surgically corrected, and foreign bodies can be removed. However, providing the epiphora is not excessive and no infection is present, the condition is often purely a cosmetic problem and does not require further treatment.

Dacryocystitis is inflammation of the nasolacrimal system and can be acute or chronic. It is more common in dogs than cats and can be caused by foreign bodies trapped in the nasolacrimal duct, such as fragments of grass seed. A purulent ocular discharge is usually present, and the eye is often uncomfortable, causing the animal to rub. The discharge is more copious at the medial canthus, and once it has been cleaned away, gently pressing below the medial canthus will often result if the appearance of more discharge from the punctum. Conjunctivitis accompanies the discharge. Samples should be taken for culture and sensitivity, and the nasolacrimal system gently flushed usually under general anaesthesia. Once patency has been established and any foreign matter removed, nursing care should include regular removal of discharge and application of topical and systemic antibiotics and anti-inflammatory agents as prescribed. Occasionally the nasolacrimal duct needs to be catheterised to re-establish patency. In this case, the catheter should be sutured in place for up to 3 weeks. During this time it is normal for the patient to wear an Elizabethan collar to prevent removing the catheter.

Reduced tear production—keratoconjunctivitis sicca M S

Keratoconjunctivitis sicca is reduced tear production, usually the aqueous component. Deficiencies of the mucous or lipid fractions are less common and will not be discussed. Keratoconjunctivitis sicca is more common in dogs than cats. Some breeds are predisposed, including English bulldogs, west Highland white terriers, cavalier King Charles spaniels and cocker spaniels (both American and English varieties). Immune-mediated cases are most common, but congenital, viral (distemper in dogs; FHV-1 in cats), drug-induced (e.g. sulphonamides), metabolic (such as hypothyroidism) and neurogenic cases all occur.

Clinical signs depend on the severity of the condition. Recurrent conjunctivitis with a mucopurulent discharge and dull, lacklustre cornea are usual. Progression leads to conjunctival hyperaemia and conjunctival thickening, corneal vascularisation and pigmentation and sometimes severe ulceration. Pain is variable but more common in acute cases. Schirmer tear test readings are diagnostic (see Chapter 3). Readings of less than 10 mm wetting in a minute confirm keratoconjunctivitis sicca, while readings of 10–15 mm are suspicious. Readings should be repeated during treatment to monitor the disease.

Treatment can be medical or surgical, and sometimes both. Medical management aims to stimulate tear production (with topical ciclosporin) and supplement tears with a variety of lubricants. These are discussed in Chapter 2. Topical antibiotics and anti-inflammatory agents might also be required. The ocular discharge needs to be removed several times during the day as it builds up, both to prevent it crusting and adhering to the eyes and to reduce the risk of bacterial contamination. Bathing with sterile saline solution is sensible. Surgical treatment in the form of parotid duct transposition is discussed in Chapter 8.

CORNEA

Corneal disease is commonly encountered in general practice. Congenital problems are rare, and most conditions are acquired. The cornea is normally transparent but will become opaque as a result of disease processes. It can only respond to pathological insults in a limited number of ways, so close ophthalmic examination is required to identify the underlying disease process. Oedema will give the cornea a blue-grey appearance, vascularisation will make it appear reddened and pigment deposition renders it darkly coloured. In general, conditions can be divided into ulcerative and non-ulcerative disease. Keratitis is the term given to corneal inflammation.

Ulcerative keratitis M S

Corneal ulceration is one of the most common ocular diseases in both dogs and cats. A sudden onset of ocular pain, with blepharospasm, increased lacrimation and photophobia is common. Examination reveals conjunctivitis and a corneal defect which is confirmed using fluorescein dye. Ulcers can be classified according to depth or cause (Table 7.4), and their management depends on both.

Simple shallow ulcers can be caused by minor trauma, including self trauma (e.g. rubbing), irritants (e.g. shampoo) and intrinsic problems, such as entropion or ectopic cilia. Removal of the cause, followed by 5 days of topical antibiotics to prevent secondary infection, will usually result in rapid healing. A single application of atropine can also be used to control ciliary spasm and promote ocular comfort.

Non-healing superficial ulcers are frequently encountered. Known also as epithelial erosion, boxer ulcer and indolent ulcer among other terms, these are very shallow, irregular ulcers, with a characteristic rim of non-adhered corneal epithelium. They can be seen in any breed, especially in middle-aged and older dogs, but are more common in boxers and corgis. With cats, both Persian and Burmese breeds are over represented. These

Table 7.4 Classification of corneal ulcers	
Classification according to depth	**Classification according to cause**
• Superficial/erosion	• Eyelash abnormality
• Shallow	• Eyelid abnormality
• Mid depth	• Irritants
• Deep	• Keratoconjunctivitis sicca
• Descemetocoele	• Trauma
• Corneal rupture/iris prolapse	• Immune-mediated
	• Infectious

ulcers can be unilateral or bilateral, and frequently recur. Many animals seem to have only mild discomfort, and the ulcers can persist for weeks or even months if not treated correctly.

Debridement of the non-adherent cornea is essential and can usually be performed under topical anaesthesia using a dry cotton bud (Fig. 7.12a). Healing can be enhanced by performing a grid keratotomy. Most ophthalmologists perform this in conscious dogs, but general practitioners tend to sedate or anaesthetise patients before the procedure. Obviously, if the patient is awake the role of the nurse in handling is vital! A fine needle is dragged across the cornea over the ulcerated area, and this stimulates healing to occur within 2 weeks (Fig. 7.12b). A bandage

contact lens can be placed to promote ocular comfort and assist healing after the procedure has been performed. A superficial non-healing ulcer is the only indication for performing a grid keratotomy—they should never be used in deeper or infected ulcers. The procedure is not usually recommended in cats since sequestrum formation can develop (p. 117). Instead, debridement and a contact lens are required. Third eyelid flaps can also be used, but the progress of the cornea cannot be monitored. Chemical cauterisation using agents such as phenol is not commonly recommended but does help if used very carefully.

Medical management with topical antibiotics to prevent secondary infection, together with lubricants and systemic NSAIDs, are also advocated. Atropine will reduce ciliary spasm and promote ocular comfort. Various other topical agents are being investigated which improve corneal wound healing, and commercial formulations will hopefully be available in future.

Deep corneal ulcers M   S

Deep ulcers, which affect more than half of the stromal depth, are serious. They require careful management to prevent the potentially disastrous progression to corneal rupture. A descemetocoele is a very deep ulcer, where only the thin layer of Descemet's membrane prevents corneal rupture. Trauma, progression from a superficial ulcer, acute keratoconjunctivitis sicca and bacterial or fungal infections can all lead to deep ulcers. Medical management revolves around treating any infectious agents (culture and sensitivity and Gram-stained samples help decide which anti-infective agent to use) and preventing a secondary uveitis. A chart should be drawn up to enable accurate recording of treatment since drops will be applied very frequently. The appearance of the eye should also be recorded when medication is applied. A melting ulcer occurs as the corneal stroma liquefies due to a combination of bacterial and autogenous collagenase activity. Management of melting ulcers is discussed in Chapter 8. Ocular lubricants will be required in ulcers caused by keratoconjunctivitis sicca and in brachycephalic breeds. In conjunction with frequent medication, surgical support is usually

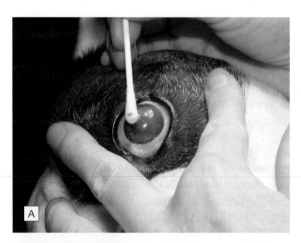

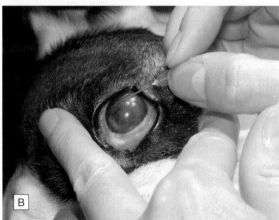

Fig. 7.12 Treatment of superficial non-healing ulcer: a) debridement of a superficial non healing ulcer; b) grid keratotomy in a 9-year-old Boston terrier.

required. The use of tissue glue, conjunctival grafts and corneoscleral transplantation is discussed in Chapter 8.

Corneal sequestrum S

Corneal sequestrum (plural, sequestra) is a condition seen in cats. Brown or black discolouration of the cornea occurs, often following ulceration or herpetic keratitis (Fig. 7.13). Persian and other brachycephalic breeds and Burmese are commonly affected, but any breed can develop the problem. A full ophthalmic examination will help identify any concomitant problems such as keratoconjunctivitis sicca, entropion or FHV-1 infection which could exacerbate the corneal disease and complicate treatment. In some cats the pigment remains in the stroma and no pain or discomfort is present. In such cases, the patients can be monitored but do not necessarily require specific treatment. However, in most cases the pigment sits as a plaque on the cornea and can look similar to an embedded foreign body. Surgical removal via superficial keratectomy with conjunctival grafting, corneoscleral transposition or contact lens placement is required (see p. 147). Nursing care will consist of topical antibiotics and lubricants for several weeks after surgery. In a few cases, if the cat is not uncomfortable, the sequestrum can be left to slough off. However, this can take months and can leave a deep ulcer or even occasionally corneal rupture, so is not usually recommended.

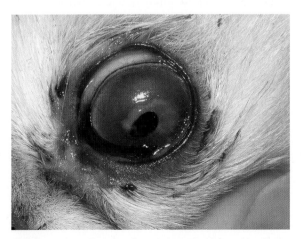

Fig. 7.13 Corneal sequestrum causing significant discomfort in a Persian cat.

It is not unusual for both eyes to be affected, and the condition can be recurrent.

Corneal injuries M S

Corneal injuries are again common in both dogs and cats. Trauma can result in superficial ulcers, deep lacerations or full thickness lacerations with iris prolapse. Obviously a careful examination of the eye and the rest of the patient is necessary to establish the extent of the injury before a treatment plan and prognosis can be reached. Deep lacerations will require surgical repair but usually heal well. Full thickness injuries are more severe since the risk of intraocular contamination is high, and panophthalmitis can result even if the corneal wound is repaired. The surgical repair of corneal injuries, including those with iris prolapse, are discussed in Chapter 8. Blunt trauma can cause severe intraocular damage, which can be difficult to assess due to hyphaema. Ocular ultrasound can assist in assessing the lens and retina for damage. If the lens has luxated or a retinal detachment is present, the visual prognosis is hopeless. Medical nursing with cool compresses, analgesics and anti-inflammatory agents are employed. Severe cases result in scleral rupture necessitating enucleation.

Corneal foreign bodies include plant material, cat claws, paint chips and metal fragments. Their depth must be carefully assessed before attempting removal. Many can be simply flushed out or lightly removed with a sterile cotton bud or ophthalmic swab. However, if the cornea is penetrated or even perforated, the surgeon must be prepared to repair the cornea once the foreign object is removed. If the equipment or expertise are not available for this, the patient should be referred. See Chapter 8 for further details.

Chemical burns constitute a medical emergency. If the nature of the agent is not known, a litmus paper strip should be dabbed onto the tear film to determine whether acid or alkali in formulation. Alkali burns (e.g. from plaster or cement dust) are generally more serious since corneal penetration occurs leading to intraocular damage. Copious irrigation with sterile saline under general anaesthesia is required until the pH returns to normal (approximately 7.5). Antibiotics and occasionally steroids are used topically to try to reduce scarring and control the associated uveitis. Referral should be considered for severe cases.

Non-ulcerative corneal disease M

Chronic superficial keratitis (pannus) is an immune-mediated condition seen most commonly in German shepherd dogs, Belgian shepherd dogs, greyhounds and lurchers. Both eyes are affected but not always symmetrically. The cornea becomes red and vascularised with plaques of granulation-type tissue ventrolaterally, and white deposits in the cornea at the leading edge of the plaque. Pigmentation also develops (Fig. 7.14). The whole cornea can be affected, leading to blindness. Nictitans plasmacytic conjunctivitis (plasmoma) can accompany the disease (p. 111). The condition is immune-mediated and can be controlled but not cured. Owners must be aware that life-long topical treatment is required. Treatment is with ciclosporin or topical steroids. Occasionally, surgery (superficial keratectomy) is required to remove the pigment and restore vision. The condition is more severe in areas with high sunlight and at higher altitudes (e.g. Australia).

Pigmentary keratitis is common in dogs but very rare in cats. It usually develops as a result of chronic low grade irritation and is prevalent in brachycephalic breeds, such as the pug. Cor-

recting the cause of irritation (medial entropion, lagophthalmos, keratoconjunctivitis sicca, etc.) will halt the progression of pigment deposition.

Crystalline stromal dystrophy manifests as bilateral corneal opacities, usually just below the central cornea. They consist of lipid deposition and are common in the Siberian husky, cavalier King Charles spaniel, rough collie and Samoyed. They do not need treatment and rarely progress, but are often noticed by owners.

Eosinophilic (proliferative) keratoconjunctivitis is an immune-mediated condition seen in cats. A white plaque or discharge is common overlying pink fleshy tissue on the corneal surface. One or both eyes can be affected. The treatment of choice is topical steroids (and occasionally ciclosporin), and long-term management is usually required (although some cats do become totally cured). Systemic medication is required in refractory cases.

THE UVEAL TRACT

The uveal tract is made up of the iris, ciliary body and choroid. In this section we will be considering the anterior uvea (i.e. the iris and ciliary body), while conditions of the choroid are mentioned later in the section on the posterior segment. In general, the uvea is highly vascular and sensitive to pathological processes. As such, it is prone to react to inflammatory and vascular conditions, such as systemic disease, and is also susceptible to traumatic damage. Like many ocular structures it can only react to noxious stimuli in a limited number of ways, and the ocular signs are similar regardless of the cause. Therefore, further laboratory investigations are frequently necessary to identify the cause for the reaction.

Congenital conditions

Congenital conditions affecting the uveal tract are limited to colour variations, lack of iris development and persistent pupillary membrane remnants.

Colour variations are quite common and are often seen with merle-coloured and colour-dilute animals (e.g. lilac point Siamese cats). If the iris in

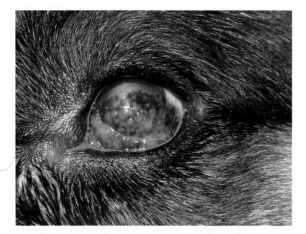

Fig. 7.14 Severe chronic superficial keratitis (pannus) in a German shepherd dog. Note also the thickening and cobblestone appearance of the third eyelid, indicating nictitans plasmacytic conjunctivitis (plasmoma).

each eye is a different colour or one is dark while the other is pale, the term heterochromia iridis is given. There is no clinical significance to the colour variations, but some owners might be concerned. Occasionally, animals with very pale irises and almost total lack of pigment are slightly photosensitive. This is because even with the pupil fully constricted light can pass through the iris tissue and stimulate the retina. However, the animals adapt by squinting or avoiding bright light, and no treatment is required apart from avoidance.

Persistent pupillary membrane remnants (PPM) are fairly common and are considered inherited in some breeds (e.g. basenji). They occur due to incomplete resorption of the vascular tissue covering the pupil which is present during embryological development. They appear as strands of tissue from the middle of the iris, which can stretch to the cornea or lens. If they attach to the lens, a small focal anterior lens capsule cataract can be present. Although they look very pretty, they are usually of no clinical concern to the animal—vision is usually unaffected (Fig. 7.15).

Acquired conditions

Uveitis M

Uveitis is inflammation of the uveal tract. Anterior uveitis affecting the iris is most common, but the ciliary body can be involved along the choroid in

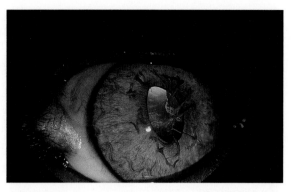

Fig. 7.15 Persistent pupillary membrane remnants in a young Burmese kitten. Note also the presence of a dermoid at the lateral canthus.

panuveitis. There are many causes for uveitis, but in general the clinical signs are similar and are listed in Table 7.5.

The causes for uveitis can be exogenous (i.e. those arising externally such as trauma) or endogenous, reaching the eye via the bloodstream (infectious, neoplastic and immune-mediated causes are the most frequent). Often the exact cause cannot be identified as the immune reaction takes over. Table 7.6 lists the more common causes for uveitis.

Further clinical investigations are usually required to try to reach a definitive diagnosis in cases of anterior uveitis. In addition to the complete ophthalmic examination, a full clinical examination is required. Blood samples are often

Table 7.5 Ophthalmic signs of anterior uveitis	
Acute signs	**Chronic signs and complications**
• Pain	• Severe ongoing pain
• Increased lacrimation	• Iris darkening
• Visual impairment	• Endophthalmitis
• Photophobia	• Cataract
• Miosis	• Lens luxation
• Aqueous flare	• Iris bombe
• Swollen iris	• Blindness
• Conjunctival hyperaemia	• Retinal detachment
• Episcleral congestion	• Glaucoma
• Corneal oedema	• Phthisis bulbi
• Lowered intraocular pressure	
• Hypopyon	
• Keratic precipitates	
• Hyphaema	
• Posterior segment changes	

Table 7.6 Common causes of uveitis

Infectious causes	Non infectious causes
Bacteria Brucellosis Lyme disease (borreliosis) Leptospirosis Bartonellosis (cats) Any septicaemia	**Immune mediated** Lens-induced (i.e. due to cataracts or lens trauma) Uveodermatological syndrome Coagulopathies, e.g. thrombocytopenia
Fungal Blastomycoses Coccidoides Cryptococcosis Histoplasmosis	**Metabolic** Diabetes mellitus (especially if cataract) Hyperlipidaemia
Viral FeLV FIV FIP Adenovirus (canine hepatitis) Distemper Rabies	**Drug induced** Excessive miotic use
Parasitic Leishmaniasis Toxoplasmosis Erlichiosis Rickettsial Migrating larvae	**Idiopathic**
Algal Prototlhecosis	**Trauma** Blunt Penetrating
	Secondary to ulceration Reflex uveitis
	Neoplastic Primary or secondary

submitted for routine haematology, biochemistry and sometimes specific diagnostic tests, such as feline leukaemia virus, leptospirosis titres or *Toxoplasma* titres. History of recent travel might make one suspicious of *Leishmania*, *Ehrlichia*, or certain fungal diseases, and these organisms should be looked for. Ocular or specific organ ultrasonography might be indicated, along with radiography and sometimes MRI. It might be necessary to take samples from the anterior chamber (paracentesis) for cytology or histology.

Treatment rests with the non-specific control of inflammation and pain, while reducing the risk of severe chronic sequelae, as well as specific medication targeting the cause whenever possible.

Most animals will receive topical corticosteroids and atropine, providing neither of these agents is contraindicated, together with systemic anti-inflammatory agents. The latter are often steroids if the condition is considered of non-infective aetiology. NSAIDs can also be used. Immunosuppressive drugs, such as azathioprine and systemic ciclosporin, are sometimes necessary, particularly for serious immune-mediated uveitis. Specific antibiotics are chosen for their ability to eliminate infectious agents (e.g. doxycycline for ehrlichiosis, penicillins for leptospirosis, clindamycin for toxoplasmosis, etc.). Severe uveitis can result in secondary glaucoma, such that enucleation is the only treatment option. Histopathology should always be performed in these cases. The eye should also be removed if neoplasia is present.

Uveal trauma M

The uveal tract can be subjected to blunt or sharp trauma. Both will cause uveitis. Blunt trauma can be severe, causing hyphaema such that ultra-sonography is required to check the rest of the eye—retinal detachments and even posterior scleral rupture can occur. Sharp trauma will lead to iris prolapse via corneal rupture (the repair of this is discussed in Chapter 8). Intraocular foreign bodies will cause a severe panuveitis.

Iris atrophy

Iris atrophy occurs as the iris degenerates, particularly the sphincter muscle, resulting in poor pupillary light reflexes and sometimes photophobia. It can be a simple ageing process (e.g. in toy breeds), or can follow uveitis, glaucoma or trauma. No specific treatment is necessary.

Iris cysts

Uveal or iris cysts are seen quite commonly in dogs and occasionally in cats. They develop from the posterior surface of the iris, which is darkly pigmented, and float through the pupil into the anterior chamber. They are usually spherical, and several can occur in one eye. Labrador retrievers and Staffordshire bull terriers seem to be particularly susceptible. They are considered to develop as an ageing change or following uveitis. On the whole, iris cysts cause no problems at all but must be differentiated from neoplasia. Some more severe types are seen in certain breeds (e.g. golden retrievers and great Danes), where cyst rupture, uveitis and glaucoma can occur.

Uveal neoplasia M   S

Although uveitis is often present with uveal tumours, this is not always the case. Neoplasia can be primary (e.g. ciliary body adenoma) or secondary (e.g. lymphoma). Melanomas are common, and there is a marked difference in the behaviour

of this tumour type between dogs and cats. In dogs, they tend to manifest as localised pigmented patches which grow slowly and are usually benign. Many do not even need treating, although laser surgery can be undertaken. In cats, uveal melanomas are more serious. They are often spread throughout the iris tissue (diffuse iris melanoma), such that surgical removal is not possible. Secondary glaucoma is quite common in these cases. Since these tumours do metastasise in cats, enucleation is usually recommended. However, they need to be differentiated from the benign pigment accumulation seen with ageing—we would not want to remove a normal eye! Cats can also develop a serious post-traumatic sarcoma. This is a highly aggressive tumour (both local invasion and metastasis) which can develop years after ocular trauma. For this reason it is sensible to advise the removal of blind traumatised eyes in this species.

Hyphaema M

Hyphaema is the presence of blood in the anterior chamber. It can be present in small amounts, associated with uveitis, or can be total such that the whole eye is filled with blood and has the appearance of a red snooker ball (Fig. 7.16). It is seen most commonly with trauma (e.g. a kick by a horse), but many other things can be causative (Table 7.7). In many cases of simple hyphaema, the blood will reabsorb, often with minimal scar-

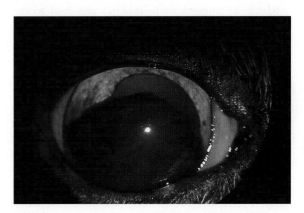

Fig. 7.16 Hyphaema in a cat with hypertension.

Table 7.7 Causes of hyphaema

General cause	Specific examples
Uveitis	FIP, erlichiosis
Trauma	Blunt or penetrating
Coagulopathies and platelet disorders	Thrombocytopenia, Von Willebrands disease, disseminated intravascular coagulation (DIC)
Systemic hypertension	Renal failure, cardiac disease
Toxins	Warfarin ingestion
Chronic glaucoma	Many causes
Neoplasia	Primary or secondary. Paraneoplastic syndromes—hyperviscosity with multiple myeloma
Congenital disease	Collie eye anomaly, persistent hyaloid artery

ring. Topical corticosteroids can be used. NSAIDs should be avoided due to their interference with platelet function. Injections of tissue plasminogen activator (tPA) can help dissolve blood clots in some cases, but these are only recommended in the hands of specialists. Sometimes secondary glaucoma can develop leading to loss of the eye.

THE LENS

Diseases of the lens can be broadly divided into cataracts (any opacity within the lens or its capsule) or lens luxation (instability and dislocation from the normal position). Other congenital conditions do occur on rare occasions and are listed in the section below. The lens is normally transparent and sits between the posterior iris and anterior face of the vitreous, held in position by fibres (called zonules, or suspensory ligaments) attached to the ciliary body (see Fig. 1.6, p. 6; and Fig. 1.9, p. 8).

Congenital conditions

Congenital lens abnormalities are quite rare in dogs, cats and horses. A total absence of the lens (aphakia) only occurs in severely malformed eyes. Microphakia, or a small lens, is slightly more common and is seen in dogs with multiple ocular abnormalities (e.g. miniature schnauzers and golden retrievers). A lens coloboma, or absence of a portion of the lens, results in a notch along the

outline of the lens and again is rarely encountered. More commonly seen are problems associated with persistent pupillary membrane (PPM) remnants and persistent hyperplastic primary vitreous (PHPV). Both of these structures represent abnormal reabsorption of the embryonic vasculature surrounding the lens, and can be present along with opacities on the anterior (with PPM) or posterior (with PHPV) lens capsules. They are not normally progressive and only affect vision if extensive and bilateral. Other forms of congenital cataract also occur from time to time. They are usually situated in the centre of the lens (nucleus), and as the animal grows, normal lens fibres form around the opacity such that the percentage of cataractous lens reduces in relation to the normal lens. In these cases, surgery is not usually necessary.

Acquired conditions of the lens

Cataract S

A cataract is an opacity of the lens or its capsule. Cataracts can be classified in several ways: the cause, the age at which the cataract appears, the position within the lens and the stage of development (Table 7.8). Inherited cataracts are commonly encountered in dogs and affect many breeds (Table 7.9 and Fig. 7.17). If the cataract has developed secondary to another ocular problem, such as uveitis or diabetes mellitus, this

Table 7.8 Different methods of classification of cataracts

Age of onset	Cause	Position	Stage of development
Congenital	Inherited	Nuclear	Incipient (very early changes with no effect on vision)
Juvenile	Secondary to other ocular disease (uveitis, generalised progressive retinal atrophy, glaucoma)	Cortical (anterior or posterior)	Immature (tapetal reflex still visible)
Senile	Trauma (blunt or penetrating)	Capsular (anterior or posterior)	Mature (entire lens opaque, eye blind)
	Metabolic (diabetes mellitus, hypocalcaemia)	Equatorial (positioned at the periphery of the lens)	Hypermature (altered density of lens and leakage from lens causing lens-induced uveitis)
	Toxic or drug induced		
	Radiation (following treatment for tumours on the head)		

Table 7.9 Inherited cataracts in dogs (UK list)

Congenital	Miniature schnauzer
Early onset with progression	Boston terrier Cavalier King Charles spaniel German Shepherd dog Leonburger Miniature schnauzer Old English sheepdog Staffordshire bull terrier Standard poodle Welsh springer spaniel
Posterior polar (upsidedown Y or triangle) Sometimes progressive	Alaskan malamute Belgian shepherd dog Chesapeake Bay retriever Golden retriever Labrador retriever Large Munsterlander Norwegian Buhund Siberian husky Staffordshire bull terrier
Other forms	American cocker spaniel Boston terrier (different from early onset cataract)
Suspected to be inherited	Many breeds including bichon frise, Border collie, Border terrier, French bulldog, giant schnauzer, Tibetan terrier, Yorkshire terrier

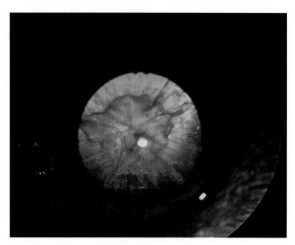

Fig. 7.17 Immature cataract in an 18-month-old golden retriever.

Table 7.10 Breeds affected by primary lens luxation

Border collie
Jack Russell terrier
Miniature bull terrier
Parson terrier
Sealyham terrier
Shar-pei
Tibetan terrier
Wire-haired fox terrier

condition needs to be treated before addressing the cataract. Some cataracts do not progress to interfere with vision, and for these no treatment is required. However, if the animal is visually disabled by the presence of cataract, surgery can be considered. Although a variety of medical agents have been advocated to slow or even prevent the progression of cataracts in humans, none to date have proven to be beneficial in controlled studies in dogs. Thus, surgery remains the only treatment for cataracts. This is discussed in Chapter 8.

Nuclear sclerosis

Nuclear sclerosis is the hardening of the lens with age. It results in a blue-grey appearance to the lens which is often confused with cataract. It is very common in middle-aged and older dogs but is only seen in very aged cats. It does not have any significant effect on vision. The easiest way to differentiate this normal change from a cataract is using distant direct ophthalmoscopy. The reflex from the fundus can be seen with nuclear sclerosis but will be broken up by the opacity if a cataract is present.

Lens luxation S

If the zonules (fibres) which hold the lens in position break, the lens can dislocate from its normal position. This is lens luxation. The condition can be primary, due to an inherited weakness in the

fibres, and occurs in terrier breeds, Border collies and occasionally the Shar Pei (Table 7.10). Secondary lens luxation in dogs can occur following glaucoma, chronic uveitis, severe trauma and sometimes cataract formation. The condition is common in cats with chronic uveitis. The lens can dislocate completely and fall into either the anterior chamber (anterior lens luxation) or into the vitreous (posterior luxation). A partially dislocated lens is called a subluxation.

Primary lens luxation is a bilateral condition and can be very serious and often blinding. The dog usually presents with one eye affected, but thorough examination of the fellow eye will often show signs of lens instability. It is seen most commonly in young adults, age 3–6 years. A dog with an acute lens luxation will have a very painful eye, and is often blind on presentation. The conjunctiva will be inflamed and corneal oedema is common, especially ventrally where the lens touches the cornea. Careful examination will reveal the presence of the lens in the anterior chamber—this can be seen from the side more clearly than from directly in front of the eye. Glaucoma is common with both anterior luxations and subluxations, and this must be treated along with removal of the lens if appropriate. Surgery for lens luxation is discussed in Chapter 8.

Secondary lens luxations do not always require surgery. If secondary to glaucoma, the lens is often subluxated, and treatment of the glaucoma is the primary concern. Uveitis will often result in luxation of the lens, especially in cats, and surgery can be successful in these cases. Any chronically luxated lens will become cataractous with time so surgical removal can be indicated to prevent blindness (providing secondary glaucoma is not present).

GLAUCOMA

Glaucoma is a raised intraocular pressure which leads to damage to the optic nerve and the retinal cells. It is a painful, often blinding condition and is a very serious disease which can be difficult to treat. There are many causes of glaucoma, and the choice of treatment often depends on the cause, the duration of disease and the potential visual outcome.

The maintenance of intraocular pressure depends on a balance between production and drainage of aqueous humour. The ciliary body produces aqueous, and it flows through the pupil into the anterior chamber and drains out of the eye through the iridocorneal angle (drainage or filtration angle). This pathway is shown in Figure 1.8 (p. 7). Most cases of glaucoma result from impaired drainage rather than from over production. Tonometry, the measurement of intraocular pressure, is essential for the diagnosis and management of glaucoma. It is impossible to diagnose and treat glaucoma successfully without the appropriate instruments, and referral to an ophthalmologist is advised should a tonometer (Schiotz or Tonopen) not be available in the surgery. In addition to measuring the intraocular pressure, gonioscopy, the examination of the iridocorneal (drainage) angle, must be performed. The techniques for both tonometry and gonioscopy are discussed in Chapter 3.

The clinical signs of glaucoma will vary pending on the cause, speed of onset, duration and how high the intraocular pressure has become (Fig. 7.18). For ease of description, the signs

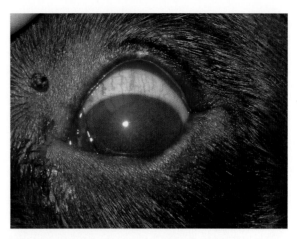

Fig. 7.18 Acute glaucoma in a 7-year-old Labrador retriever—note the episcleral congestion, corneal oedema and dilated pupil. Intraocular pressure was 36 mmHg.

are usually divided into those seen with acute glaucoma and those in chronic cases (Table 7.11).

The causes of glaucoma are broadly divided into primary and secondary. Primary glaucoma usually involves goniodysgenesis—where there is an abnormality of the drainage angle which is visible on gonioscopy (Fig. 3.17, p. 41). It is a bilateral but not usually symmetrical disease, and there can be a delay of weeks to years before the second eye is affected. Goniodysgenesis is considered inherited in several breeds, which are listed in Table 7.12. The exact relationship between the abnormal drainage angle and the development of glaucoma is unknown. Indeed, some dogs with severely malformed iridocorneal angles do not develop glaucoma at all, while others with

Table 7.11 Clinical signs of glaucoma	
Acute glaucoma	**Chronic glaucoma**
• Pain	• Enlarged globe
• Increased lacrimation	• Superficial and deep corneal vascularisation
• Blepharospasm	• Optic disc cupping (posterior bowing of optic disc from
• Protrusion of third eyelid	pressure)
• Corneal oedema	• Corneal ulceration
• Episcleral congestion	• Corneal striae (grey lines on cornea from tears in
• Dilated pupil (mydriasis)	Descemet's membrane)
• Peripheral corneal vascularisation	• Lens subluxation/luxation
• Blindness	• Retinal atrophy

Table 7.12 Breeds affected by goniodysgenesis (UK list)

American cocker spaniel
Bassett hound
Bouvier des Flandres
Dandie Dinmont terrier
English cocker spaniel
English springer spaniel
Flat coated retriever
Golden retriever
Great Dane
Labrador retriever
Siberian husky
Samoyed
Welsh springer spaniel
Welsh terrier

Table 7.13 Causes of secondary glaucoma

- Uveitis
- Lens luxation
- Cataract (intumescent or swollen, e.g. with diabetes mellitus, and hypermature)
- Hyphaema
- Intraocular neoplasia, e.g. melanoma, ciliary body adenoma
- Pigment dispersal syndrome/ocular melanosis, e.g. Cairn terrier
- Vitreal prolapse following surgical removal of the lens

relatively mild changes can have severe disease in one or both eyes. If gonioscopy reveals an abnormal angle, the animal is certainly at a higher risk from developing glaucoma than the general population, but unfortunately at present we cannot quantify this risk. The glaucoma seen with goniodysgenesis is acute and serious. The dog exhibits a sudden-onset red, cloudy, painful and often blind eye, and intraocular pressure measurement is mandatory in any of the breeds listed in Table 7.12 which present with these signs. Primary open-angle glaucoma is less common but can be encountered in the Norwegian elkhound and the beagle. Here the condition is slow in onset and vision can be maintained until quite late in the course of the disease. The increase in intraocular pressure is gradual, and the eye can tolerate these changes with less pain and globe damage than with goniodysgenesis. Congenital glaucoma is seen from time to time in all species and can affect one or both eyes.

Secondary glaucoma is encountered more frequently than primary glaucoma in both dogs and cats, as well as horses. It develops due to some other ocular abnormality leading to problems with the circulation and drainage of aqueous humour— for example, at the pupil due to adhesions between the iris and lens, or due to a tumour blocking the drainage angle. Causes of secondary glaucoma are listed in Table 7.13.

Treatment of glaucoma M S

The treatment of glaucoma can be medical or surgical, and often a combination of both is required. The medical management is discussed here, while the surgical treatment of glaucoma is a specialist procedure and discussed in Chapter 8. Reference should be made to Chapter 2 (Pharmacology and therapeutics) for an understanding of the drugs involved in treating glaucoma. The aim of treatment is to lower the intraocular pressure to a level which is comfortable and does not promote further optic nerve or retinal damage. If the eye is still visual or has the potential for a return of some vision, this will also be a major aim—to prevent a deterioration in eyesight. Unfortunately, many eyes will be irreparably blind on presentation. If the diagnosis is primary glaucoma then treatment must be targeted to prevent the same outcome for the second eye.

Emergency treatment for glaucoma should be considered in all acutely presented cases. Osmotic diuretics such as mannitol solution, are given intravenously. Care must be taken to ensure that renal function is adequate before using these agents since they can trigger renal failure in compromised patients. The pressure-lowering effect of osmotic diuretics is only short lived, and so a longer-term treatment plan involving medication or surgery must be arranged. In addition to lowering the pressure, pain relief should be provided. Long-term medication usually involves the use of topical carbonic anhydrase inhibitors, such as dorzolamine (Trusopt, MSD) and brinzolamide (Azopt, Allergan). These lower intraocular pres-

Table 7.14 Medical treatment of glaucoma

Emergency treatment	Long-term treatment
Mannitol—10–20% solution by intravenous infusion over 20–30 minutes	Topical anhydrase inhibitor, e.g. dorzolamide (Trusopt MSD)
Analgesia—systemic NSAID	Topical prostaglandin analogue, e.g. latanoprost (Xalatan, Pharmacia & Upjohn)
Paracentesis (removal of a small volume of aqueous)	Topical miotic, e.g. pilocarpine
Systemic carbonic anhydrase inhibitors, e.g. acetazolamide occasionally used	Topical beta-adrenergic blockers, e.g. timolol

sure by reducing the production of aqueous humour at the ciliary body. Topical prostaglandin analogues (such as latanoprost [Xalatan, Phamacia & Upjohn]) are used for primary glaucoma but should not be used if uveitis is present. They work by improving the outflow of aqueous, and are often used in conjunction with the topical carbonic anhydrase inhibitors. Other agents, such as miotics and beta-adrenergic blockers, are also sometimes prescribed. Table 7.14 lists some medical management options for glaucoma.

Surgery for glaucoma can include procedures to reduce the production of aqueous, such as laser and cryosurgery (cylcophotocoagulation and cyclocryotherapy, respectively), and procedures to increase outflow which involve either drainage implant surgery or scleral trephination and peripheral iridectomy. These are discussed in Chapter 8. Enucleation is also performed on many glaucomatous eyes, and this is discussed below in the section on the orbit.

THE POSTERIOR SEGMENT

The posterior segment of the eye consists of the vitreous, retina and choroid and optic disc (the latter three structures comprise the fundus).

The vitreous

The vitreous is the transparent gel which fills the posterior segment of the globe. In addition to acting as a clear medium through which light is transmitted to the retina, it provides structural support for the globe and helps to supply nutrients to and remove waste products from the retina. Conditions affecting the vitreous are not commonly encountered, and treatment specifically for the vitreous is rare. Congenital conditions do occur, most notably persistence of the hyaloid artery and persistent primary vitreous/persistent hyperplastic tunica vasculosa lentis. These three conditions are all manifestations of a lack of regression of the embryonic vasculature to the lens and can be seen as the presence of the blood vessel passing from the back of the lens to the optic disc, plaques of tissue on the back of the lens, capsular cataracts, or abnormal bowing of the posterior lens. No treatment is usually necessary (although surgical removal of the cataractous tissue and cauterisation of the blood vessel can be performed if vision is severely impaired).

Degenerative conditions of the vitreous occur following uveitis or as an ageing change. The vitreous can liquefy (syneresis) or particles of lipid–calcium complex become deposited in the vitreous gel (asteroid hyalosis). Neither condition requires treatment, although the liquefied vitreous can predispose to retinal detachment.

Occasionally, the vitreous can become infiltrated with inflammatory cells (hyalitis) as a result of generalised intraocular inflammation, and haemorrhage can occur as well.

The fundus

The fundus is the part of the posterior segment of the eye which is examined with an ophthalmoscope. It consists of the retina and choroid together with the optic disc (optic nerve head). In some animals, especially those with little pigment (e.g. merle collies), the sclera can also be seen. The retina is made up of many layers (see Chapter 1), but the photoreceptor layer, made up of rods and cones, is affected in many diseases in this part of the eye. Damage to this layer results in impaired vision or even blindness. Examination of the fundus is by indirect and direct ophthalmoscopy, providing the visual axis is clear. However, in the presence of opacification, such as cataract or hyphaema, other methods of investigation such as ultrasonography and electroretinography are required. Behavioural testing is also essential, both in bright and dim light, with obstacle courses being particularly useful.

The appearance of the normal fundus varies tremendously in dogs, but less so in cats. In most animals, the tapetum is present in the dorsal half of the fundus (the reflective layer within the choroid underlying the retina). The non-tapetal fundus makes up the rest of the area and is usually pigmented due to the presence of melanin pigment within the retinal pigment epithelium, which is the outermost layer of the retina. Thus, different colours to the tapetum, absence of the tapetum, different degrees of pigmentation in the non-tapetal fundus, various shapes to the optic disc and a range of vascular patterns are all encountered. This means that one must look at lots of eyes to be able to appreciate the wide array of normal appearance before one can appreciate what is abnormal! Ophthalmologists commonly have animals referred to them with suspected retinal haemorrhages, for example, only to find that the animal is totally normal but just lacking pigment in the fundus such that the choroidal vasculature is visible (Figs 7.19, 7.20 and 7.21 are all of a normal fundus).

Before we consider specific diseases affecting the fundus, it is important to understand the basic principles of how the area is affected by pathological processes. Abnormalities of the fundus are manifested in a limited number of ways. These are

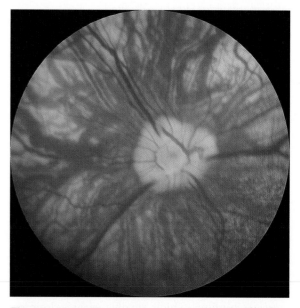

Fig. 7.20 Normal fundus appearance of a blue-merle collie.

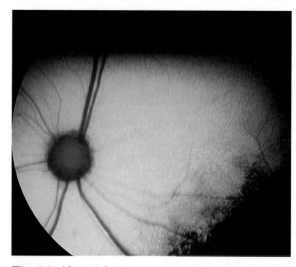

Fig. 7.21 Normal fundus appearance of a domestic short haired cat.

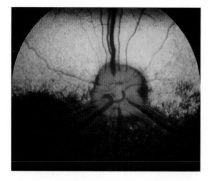

Fig. 7.19 Normal fundus appearance in a Labrador retriever.

changes in reflectivity of the tapetum, differences of pigmentation, altered vascularisation and haemorrhage. The tapetal reflex is increased (hyper-reflectivity) when the retina is thinned—more of the underlying tapetum is seen through the thinner retina. This usually signifies degeneration or atrophy of the retina. The tapetal reflex is reduced by thickening of the retina—for example, due to exudates within it, or retinal detachments. Pigmentation within the retina alters with disease; both decreased and increased amounts occur. Generally, decreased pigmentation is associated with thickening of the retina (e.g. oedema), such that the retinal pigment epithelium beneath it is less visible and hence paler. Increased pigmentation in the retinal pigment epithelium is more common and is a non-specific reaction to disease—inflammation, degeneration and injury all can cause increased pigment both in the non-tapetal and within the tapetal fundus. Changes in vascularisation can include attenuation of the retinal blood vessels (e.g. with retinal degeneration or anaemia), increased volume within the vessels making them appear thicker and more tortuous (e.g. with systemic hypertension or hyperviscosity syndromes) and blurring of the outline of the blood vessels due to inflammation and leakage (seen in active chorioretinitis). Retinal haemorrhage occurs with several diseases, and the appearance of the bleeding will vary according to which layer of the retina or choroid is affected.

Congenital disorders

Congenital disease affecting the retina and choroid occur more commonly in dogs than cats, mainly due to the incidence of inherited disorders in the former.

Collie eye anomaly (CEA)

Collie eye anomaly is a bilateral, congenital disorder in which the choroid fails to develop normally lateral to the optic disc. In affected puppies, this choroidal hypoplasia results in a pale patch of tissue in which abnormal choroidal blood vessels are present. In addition, colobomas (holes or absence of tissue) can occur on or close to the optic disc, and in a few cases retinal detachment and

intraocular haemorrhage can occur. These puppies can be blind. There is no treatment for this condition. It is common in rough and smooth collies and Shetland sheepdogs, but occurs less frequently in the Border collie. It has also been described in the Lancashire heeler and the Australian shepherd dog. The disease can be controlled by examining litters of puppies and removing those affected from the breeding pool. It is important that the animals are examined as young puppies (usually 6–8 weeks) since the abnormal lesions can become obscured with age, as the fundus matures, making accurate diagnosis in adults much more difficult. Dogs which appear funduscopically normal as adults but were visibly affected as puppies are called 'go-normals' by breeders, but obviously they are not normal. The defect has just been covered by normal tissue, and genetically they are still affected.

Retinal dysplasia

Retinal dysplasia is abnormal differentiation of the developing retina, with disorganisation and irregular proliferation of the retinal layers. Causes include inherited and non-inherited problems (Table 7.15). The breeds affected by inherited forms are numerous (Table 7.16). Several forms of the disease occur. The mildest type, focal or multifocal retinal dysplasia, manifests as small linear or circular lesions within the fundus. These appear grey in the tapetal fundus and white in the non-tapetal fundus, and represent folding of the abnormal retinal layers (often referred to as retinal folds). The more severe form of the disease, geographic retinal dysplasia, usually has larger 'folds', together with areas of retinal detachment or degeneration. These affected areas are non-functional, resulting clinically in 'blind-spots', although behaviourally

Table 7.15 Causes of retinal dysplasia

- Canine herpes virus
- Feline panleukopenia virus
- Vitamin A deficiency
- X-rays (e.g. of dam during pregnancy)
- Intrauterine trauma
- Inherited (most common form in dogs)
- Spontaneous

Table 7.16 Breed affected with inherited retinal dysplasia in the UK

Breed	Form of dysplasia
American cocker spaniel Cavalier King Charles spaniel English springer spaniel Golden retriever Hungarian Puli Labrador retriever Rottweiler	Multifocal
Cavalier King Charles spaniel English springer spaniel Golden retriever Labrador retriever	Geographic
Bedlington terrier English springer spaniel Labrador retriever Sealyham terrier	Total

affected dogs rarely show any visual problems. The most severe form of retinal dysplasia is termed total, with the retina completely detached and blindness.

In general there is no treatment for retinal dysplasia. However, if focal retinal detachments are present, laser surgery (photocoagulation) can be performed in an attempt to prevent the spread of detachment and, thus, total loss of vision.

Acquired retinal disease

Generalised progressive retinal atrophy

Generalised progressive retinal atrophy (GPRA) is a common cause of blindness in pedigree dogs and is seen occasionally in cats (Abyssinian and Siamese breeds). It is an inherited disease, most commonly as an autosomal recessive, although other forms of inheritance have been described (e.g. X-linked in the Siberian husky). The canine breeds affected in the UK are listed in Table 7.17 and the feline breeds in Table 7.18. Two main forms of the disease occur:

- *Retinal degeneration* where the photoreceptors form normally then die-away at some time after maturation.
- *Retinal or photoreceptor dysplasia* where the rods, cones or both fail to develop normally and then degenerate.

The types of GPRA seen are breed-specific, but in all cases the clinical and ophthalmological signs are similar.

Signs of GPRA which might be noted by owners include poor vision in dim light or a reluctance to go for walks in the dark, a shiny glass-like appearance to the eyes, or cataract formation. Reduced vision in dim light is a feature of rod degeneration. The eye-shine is a result of a dilated pupil and tapetal hyper-reflectivity, while the cataract development is a common finding late in the disease. Owners (and unfortunately also vets) commonly attribute the failing eyesight to the presence of the cataract rather than the primary underlying retinal degeneration.

Ophthalmological signs include dilated pupils with slow incomplete pupillary light reflexes (although this finding is not consistent), tapetal hyper-reflectivity, blood vessel attenuation and optic disc atrophy (Fig. 7.22). Total retinal degeneration develops. Reduced pigment in the non-tapetal fundus develops along with secondary cataracts, as mentioned above.

There is no treatment for this condition and affected dogs become totally blind. The time taken for this to occur varies between breeds, and even between affected dogs from the same litter. Owners must be educated how to interact with their blind pet, and nurses can be very helpful in this respect. The condition is slow in onset, giving the animal

Table 7.17 Canine breeds with generalised progressive retinal atrophy in the UK

Breed	Age at which ophthalmoscopic signs visible
Australian cattle dog	> 6 years (quite variable)
Collie (rough)	4 months
Dachshund (miniature long haired)	5 months
Elkhound	12 months
Finnish lapphund	3 years (approx)
Irish setter	4 months
Irish wolfhound	9 months (sometimes earlier)
Lhasa apso	3 years +
Miniature schnauzer	12 months
Poodle (miniature and toy)	3 years
Retriever (Chesapeake Bay)	8 months early onset, 4 years later onset
Retriever (Golden)	3 years
Retriever (Labrador)	4 years
Retriever (Nova Scotia duck tolling)	3 years
Spaniel (American cocker)	3 years
Spaniel (cocker)	3 years
Spaniel (English springer)	12 months
Tibetan spaniel	12 months
Tibetan terrier	12 months
Welsh corgi (cardigan)	3 months

Table 7.18 Feline breeds with generalised progressive retinal atrophy

Breed	Age at onset (ophthalmic signs)
Abyssian	Dominant form at 8 weeks Recessive form at 18–24 months
Siamese	8–10 years

plenty of time to adjust to its disability, and quality of life remains very good. Further information on living with a blind pet is found in Chapter 4.

Retinal pigment epithelial dystrophy (RPED)

This is a second form of retinal degeneration, which is also called central progressive retinal atrophy (CPRA). Like GPRA, it is considered inherited,

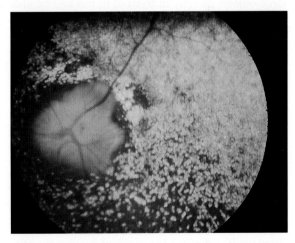

Fig. 7.22 Generalised progressive retinal atrophy in an 11-year-old poodle.

Table 7.19 Breeds with retinal pigment epithelial dystrophy in the UK

- Border collie
- Briard
- Collie (rough and smooth)
- Retriever (golden and Labrador)
- Shetland sheepdog
- Spaniel (cocker and English springer)
- Welsh corgi (cardigan)

and some breeds suffer from both forms of degeneration. Affected breeds are listed in Table 7.19, but the specific mode of inheritance is not fully understood. The disease can be considered an ophthalmic manifestation of a systemic disease since affected animals have very low Vitamin E levels. Supplementation with Vitamin E can often halt progression of the disease, although the damaged cells do not regenerate. As the name suggests, it is the cells of the retinal pigment epithelial layer which are primarily affected, and the photoreceptors become involved later on.

Affected animals suffer from a slowly progressive reduction in central vision. Owners might perceive this in the dog as an ability to see a ball thrown from the side but not when thrown directly in front. Similarly, the dog might run into large objects directly in front of it, but still be able to chase a moving fly. Animals are usually over 18–24 months of age before signs become apparent. If not diagnosed early, the disease can progress to total blindness, although this is not as inevitable as it is with GPRA. Neurological signs can develop in some dogs, associated with the low vitamin E levels (English cocker spaniels in particular). Ataxia and hind limb weakness are initially seen.

Ophthalmoscopic signs of RPED include patches of brown discolouration in the tapetal fundus, starting laterally then progressing to include all of the tapetal area. Later in the course of the disease, more advanced retinal degeneration can develop. If a dog is suspected of having the disease, it is essential to measure plasma vitamin E levels. If these are reduced, supplementation with high levels of a natural source of vitamin E is recommended.

Sudden acquired retinal degeneration (SARD)

Sudden acquired retinal degeneration (SARD) is seen in dogs and, as the name suggests, affected animals become blind very quickly, usually over 1–2 days (occasionally it can take a couple of weeks). Owners tend to notice their pet bumping into things or being quiet and withdrawn. Some dogs also have increased appetite, polydipsia and polyuria. On examination, pupils are usually widely dilated and non-responsive, but the fundus initially looks normal. It is only after a few weeks that degeneration becomes visible (with tapetal hyper-reflectivity, blood vessel attenuation and optic disc atrophy). If SARD is suspected, blood samples should be taken for routine haematology, biochemistry and ACTH stimulation tests, since some dogs are shown to have Cushing's disease. A definitive diagnosis of SARD can be made by electroretinography (see Chapter 3). This electro-diagnostic test will also differentiate the disease from optic neuritis or central causes of blindness (discussed below). Unfortunately, there is no treatment for SARD and affected animals remain blind. Although initially this can be quite distressing, they do adapt within a few weeks and can lead near-normal lives in spite of not seeing. Chapter 4 (Medical nursing) provides further information for client education on dealing with a permanently blind pet.

Retinal detachment M S

Detachments of the retina occur for a variety of reasons, and the effect on vision varies from minimal to complete blindness. Small areas can detach due to accumulation of fluid beneath the retina (serous or exudative detachments), and these can coalesce resulting in a total detachment (Fig. 7.23). Retinal tears are quite common (e.g. following trauma, including intraocular surgery) and often result in blindness. Traction detachments are also encountered, where fibrosis or inflammation within the vitreous leads to bands of tissue pulling the retina from its attachments. A thorough ophthalmic examination is required to try to elucidate the cause of the detachment (e.g. chorioretinitis, hypertension or hypermature cataracts). Medical treatment is used for some

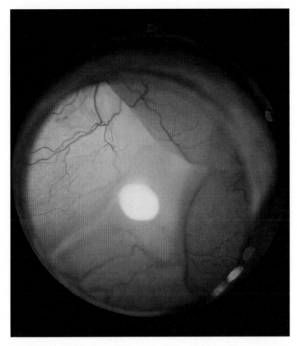

Fig. 7.23 Total retinal detachment in a cat with hypertension.

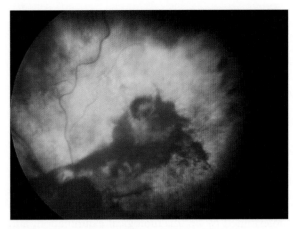

Fig. 7.24 Hypertensive retinopathy in an elderly cat.

types of detachment (e.g. immune-mediated detachments in the German shepherd dog), while sometimes laser surgery can be employed to weld the retina back into position (see Chapter 8).

Hypertensive retinopathy M

Hypertension is common in both cats and dogs. It is often secondary to systemic problems, such as renal insufficiency, cardiac disease or hyperthyroidism, and a complete physical examination and diagnostic work-up is required in all cases. Primary hypertension, where no underlying dis-

ease can be established, can occur but less frequently. Affected animals can present in a variety of ways. Sudden-onset blindness occurs due to retinal detachment (Fig. 7.23), and the owner may notice the dilated pupils or change in appearance of the eyes. Haemorrhages are common, both into the vitreous and the anterior chamber, and the owner will be aware of the colour change (Fig. 7.16). Bleeding into the posterior segment can appear very dark, almost black in colour, and the owner might notice that the eye has lost its shiny appearance. Fundus examination of affected patients might also reveal small areas of retinal haemorrhages, blood vessel tortuosity and blister-like retinal detachments (bullous retinopathy) (Fig. 7.24). Measurement of systolic blood pressure will assist diagnosis (see Chapter 3 for further details). Treatment of the underlying disease, if present, together with specific anti-hypertensive agents (Table 7.20) can restore or improve vision in many cases. However, retinal degeneration often

Table 7.20 Treatment for hypertension

Drug name	Class of drug	Method of action
Amlodipine Diltiazem	Calcium-channel blocker	Stabilise heart rate and vasodilate
Enalapril Benazepril	Angiotensin-converting enzyme (ACE) inhibitor	Vasodilation to reduce cardiac workload
Propranolol	Beta-blocker	Reduces heart rate
Frusemide	Diuretic	Reduces extracellular fluid volume

develops in spite of an initial encouraging response, and owners must be aware that their pet is quite likely to eventually lose all sight.

Chorioretinitis M

Chorioretinitis is inflammation of the choroid and retina. It can occur alone or with anterior segment inflammation as well (panophthalmitis). There are numerous causes, including viruses (e.g. canine distemper and feline panleukopenia), generalised septicaemia, toxoplasmosis, parasites (e.g. *Toxocara*) and fungal diseases. The cause cannot be determined by ophthalmological examination, and thus a thorough diagnostic work-up with a full clinical examination, blood tests, radiography and so on is required. Sometimes only one eye is affected, although more commonly both are involved but not usually in a symmetrical pattern (unlike the inherited retinal diseases). Since the animal might present with a systemic illness, it is important to check the eyes—they might not be presented because of visual problems.

The fundus appearance of chorioretinitis varies according to whether the condition is active or inactive. With the former, areas of inflammatory cell infiltrates will appear as greyish patches, often following the path of the blood vessels. Haemorrhages might also be seen together with retinal detachment. Later on the affected areas become degenerate and appear as hyper-reflective regions, often with darkly pigmented centres. These are termed post-inflammatory retinopathy. If large areas of the fundus are affected, blindness can ensue.

The prognosis for chorioretinitis obviously depends on the cause and severity, as well as choice of appropriate medical therapy. In addition to specific treatment (clindamycin for toxoplasmosis, oxytetracyclines for erlichiosis, etc.), anti-inflammatory agents might be required. However, care must be exercised with the use of systemic steroids if an infectious aetiology is present.

Taurine deficiency in cats M

A form of retinal degeneration is occasionally encountered in cats, associated with low dietary levels of the amino acid, taurine. This is an essential amino acid for cats, as they cannot manufacture it themselves unlike dogs and other species. Thus, cats fed dog food, for example, will not have sufficient levels unless supplemented. Feline central retinal degeneration is the name given to the ophthalmic changes—initially a lateral patch of tapetal hyper-reflectivity which can progress through several stages to a total retinal degeneration and blindness. Supplementation with taurine will halt progression but not reverse the changes already present. Some cats with taurine deficiency have cardiac disease (dilated cardiomyopathy), and thus a full cardiac assessment is necessary. Conversely, cats presented with a cardiomyopathy should have their eyes examined and taurine levels measured!

Other retinal diseases

Several other changes can be seen on fundus examination where systemic disease is present. These include anaemia, hyperviscosity syndromes, hypercholesterolaemia and other lipid abnormalities and coagulopathies. Thus, a full ophthalmic examination is required in many medical conditions—something which unfortunately is often overlooked in general practice.

OPTIC NERVE M

Diseases affecting the optic nerve are not common. Congenital conditions include a small optic disc (micropapilla if vision is present and optic nerve hypoplasia if the affected eye is blind). Some breeds of dog, such as the miniature and toy poodles, may have an inherited tendency for this. Colobomas (holes) in the optic disc are seen in association with collie eye anomaly and as a sporadic finding in any breed, as well as very occasionally in cats.

Acquired diseases of the optic nerve include swelling of the disc (papilloedema) seen with raised intracranial pressure, and inflammatory changes including the swelling, haemorrhage and blindness seen with optic neuritis. In addition to a general clinical examination and laboratory investigation, a neurological assessment is essential with any animals which have optic disc swelling. Further diagnostic tests, such as cerebrospinal fluid analysis and MRI, might be required to reach a definitive diagnosis. Causes of papilloedema and optic neuritis include central neoplasia, granulomatous meningoencephalitis and immune-mediated conditions. Atrophy of the optic disc will occur with severe retinal degeneration and following optic neuritis, while 'cupping' of the disc (a backward bowing) is seen in glaucoma. Tumours affecting the optic disc are rare.

ORBIT M S

Diseases affecting the orbit occur quite commonly in dogs and cats, and also in rabbits (discussed separately later in this chapter). The orbit is the region containing the eye, extraocular muscles, lacrimal glands, optic nerve and other nerves supplying the area, and associated blood vessels. The structures are contained mostly within bone, although there is soft tissue, mainly along the ventral wall of the orbit. (Fig. 1.1, p. 2). The close relationship to the nasal chamber, frontal and maxillary sinuses, and molar tooth roots mean that conditions affecting these tissues can also extend to include orbital signs. In addition, disease processes in the masticatory muscles and salivary glands can cause orbital disease.

The clinical signs of orbital disease tend to be similar regardless of the cause and are listed in Table 7.21. Thus exophthalmos, the protrusion of the globe with elevation of the third eyelid, is the most consistent findings. Localised swelling, squint (strabismus), pain on opening the mouth, chemosis (swelling of the conjunctiva) and conjunctivitis can all be present. The patient might suffer from lagophthalmos (inability to fully blink), which can result in corneal ulceration. Generalised systemic signs

Table 7.22 Causes of retrobulbar disease

Common conditions	Less common conditions
• Retrobulbar abscess • Retrobulbar cellulitis • Masticatory myositis (dog) • Neoplasia	• Retrobulbar foreign body • Lacrimal gland cysts • Salivary gland cysts • Extraocular muscle myositis • Arteriovenous shunts • Retrobulbar haemorrhage

can include pyrexia, general malaise and reduced appetite.

Differential diagnoses for orbital disease are listed in Table 7.22. In addition to the clinical signs, the history is important in establishing the aetiology. For example, a sudden onset of unilateral exophthalmos with general malaise and pain on opening the mouth in a young dog might suggest an abscess or cellulitis, while a slowly progressive, non-painful exophthalmos with an outward squint in an elderly cat is more indicative of neoplasia, perhaps extending from the nasal chambers. Figure 7.25a shows a cat with severe exophthalmos and third eyelid protrusion of the left eye. This was due to a tooth root abscess, and the same cat is shown 24 hours later after a dental in Figure 7.25b and looks significantly improved already. Sometimes it can be difficult to distinguish between a true exophthalmos, where the globe is displaced anteriorly, and an enlarged globe due to chronic glaucoma. Obviously, there will be multiple ophthalmic changes in the glaucomatous eye, but another simple way to tell the difference is to look at the patient from above. The exophthalmic eye will protrude forwards while the glaucomatous one will be in the same plane as the fellow eye, just enlarged. A further clue to the nature of the problem is provided by retropulsion, the gentle pushing of the eye back into the socket through the closed eyelids. There will be resistance to this and often pain or discomfort in cases of orbital disease. The amount that the globe will move backward depends also on the breed. In brachycephalics and cats there is little movement, whereas in breeds like the

Table 7.21 Ophthalmic signs of orbital disease

- Exophthalmos
- Protrusion of the third eyelid (nictitans membrane)
- Squint (strabismus)
- Periorbital swelling
- Conjunctival hyperaemia
- Lagophthalmos
- Corneal ulceration
- Pain on opening mouth

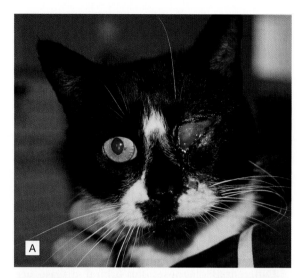

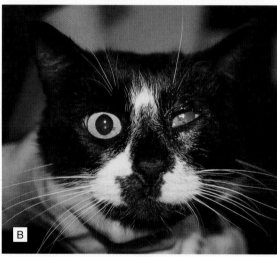

Fig. 7.25 Exophthalmos: a) cat showing exophthalmos of the left eye due to dental disease; b) same cat 24-hours later (after treatment).

rottweiler and spaniels the eye can be pushed back a couple of centimetres.

In addition to the ophthalmic and general clinical examination, diagnostic imaging is often employed with the investigation of orbital disease. Ultrasonography is performed in conscious patients with topical anaesthesia, while general anaesthesia is required for skull radiography, CT and MRI.

Retrobulbar abscesses and cellulitis are quite common in both dogs and cats, and can be associated with trauma, tooth root infections and foreign bodies. Management usually includes both medical and surgical approaches. Thus, broad-spectrum antibiotics and anti-inflammatory agents are given systemically, together with topical ophthalmic lubricants or antibiotic ointments to reduce corneal drying leading to ulceration. Surgical drainage of the abscess is attempted via the mouth. Under general anaesthesia (with a cuffed endotracheal tube and packing the back of the mouth to prevent aspiration of discharge), an incision is made behind the last molar on the affected side. Gentle probing with a blunt instrument towards the retrobulbar space can yield purulent material. Swabs should always be taken for culture and sensitivity, even if little discharge seems present.

Neoplasia of the orbital region tends to be serious. Many tumour types are possible, but carcinomas extending from the nasal chambers and fibrosarcomas are common and the prognosis is guarded. Biopsy samples should be obtained when possible. If surgical exploration is to be considered, thorough imaging with CT or MRI is essential to delineate the tumour such that a surgical plan can be made. Often the globe has to be removed to access the tumour.

Other less common orbital diseases include masticatory muscle myositis, extraocular muscle myositis and salivary gland mucocoeles.

Enophthalmos (the inward sinking of the eye) can occur with some orbital disease. This can be mistaken for a small or shrunken eye. Pain will make the eye retract into the orbit, as will atrophy of the orbital tissues (e.g. in elderly cats) and some neurological conditions such as Horner's syndrome (disruption of the sympathetic supply to the eye). Microphthalmos is a small eye which is congenital and can be found sometimes in both dogs and cats. Some pedigree dogs are bred for a small eye (e.g. rough collies). Some microphthalmic eyes are normally developed but just small, while others can be part of the multiple ocular abnormality complex and have cataracts, retinal dysplasia and nystagmus, for example.

Prolapse of the globe S

Prolapse of the globe (proptosis) is unfortunately quite common, particularly in brachycephalic

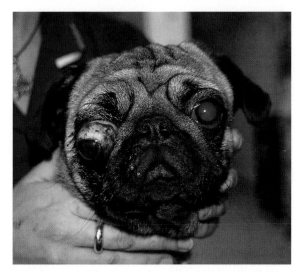

Fig. 7.26 Traumatic proptosis of the right eye in a pug.

breeds (Fig. 7.26). Here the shallow orbit and relative lack of protection to the eye make it very easy for minimal trauma to result in forward displacement of the eye, such that the lids close behind it. More severe trauma, such as road traffic accidents and dog fights, can result in proptosis in other breeds and cats. Here the eye is often seriously traumatised and irreparably damaged.

Proptosis is an emergency. The treatment plan is detailed in Table 7.23. Initial advice to give to owners should include protecting the exposed eye and keeping it moist. Thus the use of a damp cloth over the eye or a water-based lubricant such as KY jelly (Johnson & Johnson) should be advised. A full clinical examination of the patient should be made prior to anaesthesia. Victims of road traffic accidents might have other, more serious, injuries which need attention. Following proptosis, the eyelids rapidly go into spasm behind the globe such that pressure on the eye will not result in its return to a normal position. By incising through the lateral canthus (lateral canthotomy) under general anaesthesia and placing sutures through the lids, they can be pulled out and over the globe, while gently pushing the eye back into the socket. Severe swelling and haemorrhage will mean that the eye is unlikely to sit in its normal position. Prior to suturing the lids together, a third eyelid flap can be placed to help secure the eye in position, but often there is too much swelling present to allow this. The sutures are left in place for 1–2 weeks while the patient receives topical antibiotic ointment through the sutures and systemic antibiotic and anti-inflammatory agents.

Table 7.23 Checklist for proptosis

Activity	Action
Owner advice	• Prevent self trauma • Keep eye moist with damp cloths or lubricating ointment • Attend surgery as soon as possible
Initial assessment	• Gently clean proptosed globe with sterile saline • Gently attempt to reposition (rarely successful) • Assess degree of extraocular damage—to muscles and optic nerve • Check pupillary light reflex if possible (any reaction in affected eye or consensual to the fellow eye is encouraging) • Fluorescein stain cornea for ulceration • Check patient for suitability for anaesthesia
Surgery	• Clean and prep patient for surgery • Get suitable surgical kits and suture material • Assist surgeon in replacing globe or enucleation if damage too severe for attempts at salvage • Recover patient from anaesthesia
Post operative care	• Nurse patient during recovery • Ensure adequate pain relief • Draw up treatment plan according to VS instructions

Once the sutures are removed the eye can be assessed. Often a lateral squint will be present and many eyes remain blind. However, if the patient is comfortable and can blink properly, an acceptable cosmetic result can be achieved. Unfortunately, some eyes will require enucleation.

Other orbital trauma is occasionally encountered, including fractures following road traffic accidents or being kicked by a horse or shotgun injuries. The prognosis in these cases will clearly depend on the degree of damage to the eye and surrounding structures.

Enucleation S

Enucleation is the surgical removal of the globe. It is necessary for several severe ophthalmic problems. These include extensive ocular trauma, proptosis where the optic nerve or extraocular muscles have all been ruptured, intraocular neoplasia, unmanageable glaucoma and any other permanently blind, painful eye. Owners might initially be reluctant to have their pet's eye removed. However, with counselling and reassurance that the cosmetic outcome is not unsightly (Fig. 7.27),

owners usually agree that it is in the best interests of their pet to have the surgery performed.

The management plan for enucleation is outlined in Table 7.24. The procedure is performed under general anaesthesia. Two main approaches are used. The sub-conjunctival approach involves removing the eye first by cutting around the conjunctiva and then dissecting close to the globe, ligating the retrobulbar vessels and then removing the eyelids, third eyelid and any remaining conjunctiva. Haemorrhage should be fully controlled before closing the orbital fissure. This is done using two layers of absorbable sutures, and then the skin is sutured with non-absorbable material.

The second approach, the transpalpebral approach, entails removing the eyelids at the same time as the globe. The eyelids are sutured together and are excised along with the eyeball. This results in more bleeding, but it can be easier to manipulate the globe during removal. This technique is preferred if there are neoplastic or infectious processes which could have spread beyond the globe itself. Histology of the enucleated globe should always be considered. An alternative to enucleation is the implanting of a silicone prosthesis into the sclera once the intraocular contents have been removed. This technique is more common in the USA and Australia than in the UK, and is discussed in Chapter 8.

OCULAR SIGNS OF SYSTEMIC DISEASE

Ocular signs are quite common with a variety of systemic diseases. Therefore, a full general clinical examination should be performed if suspicious ocular signs are seen and, conversely, medical patients should have a thorough ocular examination. A detailed description of all potential diseases and their ocular manifestations is beyond the scope of this book. Needless to say, infectious (bacterial, viral, fungal, parasitic and protozoan), endocrine (diabetes mellitus, hypothyroidism, hyperadrenocorticism), neoplastic (lymphoma and any metastatic disease), haematologic (anaemia, thrombocytopenia, hyperviscosity syndromes) and various other disease processes can all include ocular signs. In general, if the patient is systemically unwell with bilateral ocular disease, a thorough clinical investigation is warranted.

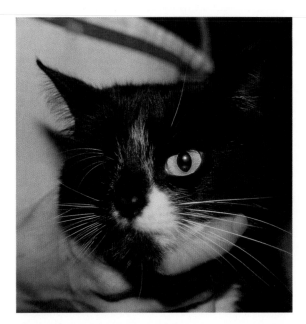

Fig. 7.27 Appearance of a cat following enucleation of the right eye.

Table 7.24 Treatment plan for enucleation

Activity	Action
Owner counselling prior to surgery	• Discuss procedure with owner on admission • Explain how the patient will look following surgery, showing photographs of other animals immediately after surgery and once the fur has grown back • Reassure owner that patient will be more comfortable once eye removed • Follow standard admission procedure
Surgery	• Prepare patient for surgery • Prepare theatre • Prepare surgical instruments including suture materials • Check if surgeon requires additional items (e.g. extra swabs, haemostatic agents) • Assist surgeon during procedure if required • Recover patient from surgery
Postoperative	• Draw-up treatment plan for patient • Start postoperative medication as instructed • Fill out discharge instructions for owner • Discuss with owner what to expect in days following surgery and what to be concerned about, e.g. minor oozing from the wound is acceptable for 12 hours post surgery but veterinary attention should be sought if any significant bleeding or epistaxis occur

OCULAR EMERGENCIES

For details of genuine ocular emergencies please refer to Appendix 1.

OPHTHALMIC CONDITIONS IN RABBITS

Rabbits are very popular as pets nowadays and as a result present with a wide variety of veterinary problems. They do suffer from ocular problems quite frequently and an understanding of some of these conditions is important for nurses.

A commonly seen problem in rabbits is dacryocystitis or infection and inflammation of the nasolacrimal ducts. It can affect one or both eyes and typically presents as a milky-white ocular discharge which can be copious. Matting of the fur around the medial canthus can occur, and if allowed to accumulate the eyelids can become stuck together from the discharge. Material should be collected for culture and sensitivity. *Pasteurella multocida* is a common pathogen in rabbits, but other bacteria, including *E. coli* and staphylococcal species, also occur. Repeated nasolacrimal flushes are usually recommended, in addition to systemic and topical antibiotics (e.g. systemic enfloxacin and topical fusidic acid, both of which are licensed for use in rabbits in the UK). The rabbit only has one ventral nasolacrimal punctum, which can usually be easily cannulated in the conscious animal following topical anaesthesia. Flushing with sterile saline is attempted. The nasolacrimal duct in rabbits is very long and twisting, with different diameters along its length and, as such, blockages frequently occur, either where the duct bends or where it narrows. Dental problems can also impinge on the nasolacrimal duct causing blockages (the duct runs close to the roots of the incisors and molars). Patience and gentle pressure can sometimes free the blockage, but in longstanding cases there may be permanent occlusion. Long-term oral antibiotics might be required, along with frequent cleansing of the ocular discharge. Rabbits can live quite happily despite the unpleasant discharge, providing they do not have any ocular discomfort (e.g. from conjunctivitis or ulceration).

A second, regularly encountered rabbit eye problem is the retrobulbar abscess. Again *Pasteur-*

ella multocida is a frequent quoted pathogen, and extension from dental disease is commonly implicated. The condition is serious and can be life-threatening. Surgical drainage is difficult, and a combined approach with dental extraction, enucleation and curettage of the abscess can be employed. If enucleation is required, care must be taken to avoid the retrobulbar venous plexus, a group of large blood vessels from which there can be serious (even life-threatening) bleeding if the surgical approach is not meticulous.

Other ocular problems are seen less frequently. Conjunctivitis can occur due to irritation (e.g. dust from poor quality bedding). Bacterial conjunctivitis should be treated aggressively with topical antibiotics and regular bathing to reduce the risk of spread to the nasolacrimal ducts. Myxomatosis is common in wild rabbits, with the acute periocular swelling and facial oedema being classic symptoms. A rare but strange condition seen from time to time is that of aberrant conjunctival overgrowth. A membrane of conjunctiva grows over the cornea in a circular pattern from the limbus and affects vision if severe and bilateral. Surgical removal will only provide a temporary cure (the fold of tissue will grow back), unless the cut edge is sutured to the sclera to force it to stay in position. Corneal ulcers occur in the same way as in dogs and cats. Some require surgery to achieve healing. Cataracts (Fig. 7.28) uveitis and glaucoma also occur in rabbits, and treatment options are similar to those for dogs and cats. However, care must be exercised with some medications since they are not licensed for use in this species and systemic side-effects can occur.

Medicating rabbits

General nursing for ocular problems in rabbits includes bathing the eyes regularly to prevent a build-up of discharge, as mentioned above for dacryocystitis. Topical administration of both drops and ointments is quite easy in rabbits. If the patient is not used to being handled or is nervous, it should be wrapped in a towel to reduce the risk of injury. Since the eyes are positioned laterally, it is usually easier to apply drops from above, lifting the upper lid and placing a drop onto the dorsal conjunctiva or cornea. Ointments can be placed onto the conjunctiva in the same way. Rabbits can rub with their front feet or rub up against bedding and cage walls, and sometimes an Elizabethan collar is required to prevent self trauma. It is important to ensure that they can still eat and drink while wearing the collar.

SMALL AND EXOTIC ANIMALS

Other small animals, such as rats, mice, gerbils and hamsters, all can suffer from ocular problems. These are similar in principle to the conditions discussed above, but most commonly involve conjunctivitis and corneal ulceration associated with irritants such as straw dust or foreign bodies. The ocular discharge often sticks these tiny eyes together, and regular bathing is required prior to administering medication. Ointments tend to attract further debris (e.g. sawdust), and so gels or drops are preferred. A dust-free bedding such as shredded paper should be considered until the eyes are back to normal.

Birds kept as pets or in wildlife sanctuaries are occasionally presented with eye problems. Localised swellings associated with sinus problems are common. Viruses, bacteria and parasites can cause blepharitis and conjunctivitis. Corneal ulcers can be treated with third eyelid flaps. Uveitis and trauma

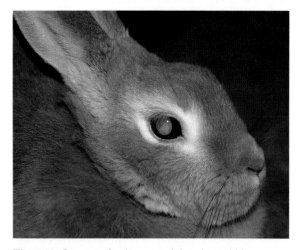
Fig. 7.28 Cataract of unknown aetiology in a rabbit.

can be blinding. Birds which are bilaterally blind (e.g. due to cataracts) often fail to feed, and as such phacoemulsification is occasionally performed.

Reptiles can suffer from diet-related ocular problems—a lack of vitamin A will cause swelling of the eyelids and keratoconjunctivitis sicca in tortoises and other reptiles. Thus, questions about husbandry must be considered in all patients presented with eye conditions. Snakes can suffer from retained spectacles—these are the transparent parts of their skin which overlie the cornea. They should be shed along with the rest of the skin. If retained, they become opaque and can trap infections. Gentle bathing with a wet cotton bud will sometimes loosen the tissue, but it may be necessary to wait until the next skin slough. All species can suffer from trauma, causing a range of symptoms from corneal ulceration, hyphaema, cataract formation and even prolapse of the eyeball.

BIBLIOGRAPHY AND FURTHER READING

Gelatt KN, Gelatt JP. Handbook of small animal ophthalmic surgery. Volumes 1 and 2. Oxford: Pergamon; 1994.

Gelatt KN. Veterinary ophthalmology. 3rd edn. Philadelphia: Lippincott Williams & Wilkins; 1999.

Grahn B, Cullen C, Peiffer R. Veterinary ophthalmology essentials. Oxford: Butterworth-Heinemann; 2004.

Petersen-Jones S, Crispin S, eds. BSAVA manual of small animal ophthalmology. 2nd edn. Gloucester: British Small Animal Veterinary Association; 2002.

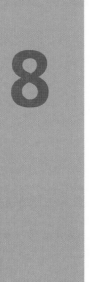

8 Specialist ophthalmic procedures

INTRODUCTION

In this chapter we will review specialist ophthalmic procedures, the majority of which are surgical. Normally, these procedures will be undertaken by specialist ophthalmologists in referral ophthalmic practice and not by general practitioners. We will follow the same format as the previous chapter, such that we start in the front of the eye and work our way through to the back of the eye. It is important to refer to the chapters on anatomy, surgical nursing and general ophthalmic conditions while reading this chapter. The role of the nursing team is vital to the success of these specialist procedures, and a well-trained nurse who understands the procedures and the reason why certain protocols are followed will greatly assist the smooth-running of events.

COMPLEX EYELID SURGERY

Although many eyelid procedures can be performed in general practice (e.g. the correction of simple entropion or the removal of a small eyelid tumour), more complicated procedures should be referred to an ophthalmologist. For example, a Saint Bernard or great Dane with 'diamond eye', where there is a combination of upper lid entropion, lower lid entropion and ectropion, and instability of the lateral canthus, poses a challenge to correct. Figure 8.1 shows an 8-month-old dogue de Bordeaux with similar problems—he has a combination of dreadful eyelid conformation and a prolapsed nictitans gland in the left eye. His eyes are so deep-set that they cannot be seen. Correction of these multiple problems to create as near normal anatomy as possible is clearly a specialist procedure, and for this type of dog more than one surgical procedure is likely to be required. Nursing duties will include client education. The surgery is likely to alter the appearance of their pet

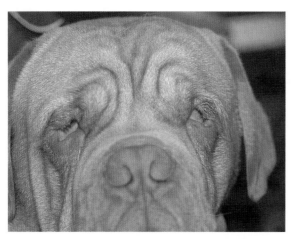

Fig. 8.1 Dogue de Bordeaux with poor eyelid conformation and prolapsed nictitans gland in the left eye.

and owners might be resistant to this, despite the fact that the dog has very sore eyes and cannot see! A whole variety of complicated surgical procedures has been described to correct this type of conformational problem, and the surgeon will have decided on which method best suits each individual patient.

For any complex eyelid surgery, it is essential that the patient is carefully prepared for surgery. This might include preoperative systemic antibiotics for several days before surgery, as skin infections and wound breakdown should be avoided. Gentle but thorough clipping of the hair is needed, which can be difficult in certain breeds with spiky fur, such as the Shar-pei, or those with abundant loose skin, such as the bloodhound. It is necessary to take plenty of time to clip and disinfect the area properly once the patient is anaesthetised. In general, the surgeon will require an extraocular kit, together with a scalpel blade, plenty of swabs and several packets of suture material—the choice of this will depend on surgeon preference, the breed and the procedure being performed. For major lid surgery, electrocoagulation might be required, either with a hand-held cautery unit (shown in Fig. 5.5, p. 66) or a general surgery unit.

In addition to conformational correction, specialised surgery on the eyelids might include the removal of large eyelid tumours or the correction of eyelid colobomas. For this type of procedure,

sliding or rotating skin flaps lined with conjunctiva are employed to recreate the palpebral fissure.

Rhytidectomy (face lift)

Certain breeds of dog suffer from upper lid entropion as a result of a heavy brow and multiple skin folds sinking down over the eyes. The chow chow and Shar-pei spring to mind! In these cases a 'face lift' or rhytidectomy is required. The instruments required for this procedure are listed in Table 8.1. This is major surgery, and large amounts of redundant skin are removed to lift the upper lids back to a more normal position. The position and shape of the skin to be removed depends very much on the individual's conformation. A horizontal band from behind the ears, a star-shaped resection or an ellipse of tissue from between the ears might be removed. A sterile marker pen is used to outline the area for resection. Meticulous suturing of both the subcutaneous tissue and skin is necessary, including anchoring the subcutaneous tissue to the underlying periosteum of the skull to prevent further slippage over time. Often surgical drains need to be placed for a couple of days after the surgery, and these require regular nursing attention. For details of the nursing requirements with surgical drains, refer to a standard nursing text. An Elizabethan collar is worn until the skin sutures are removed, usually 14 days postoperatively.

Before any surgery is undertaken, the owners need to be aware that the procedure will change the appearance of their pet, but once the wrinkles

---

Table 8.1 List of equipment required for rhytidectomy (face-lift procedures)

- Vacuum cushion for positioning
- General surgical kit
- Surgical drapes
- Sterile marker pen
- No. 15 or 10 Bard-Parker scalpel blade
- Electrocautery unit
- Sterile swabs (standard size)
- Suture material—absorbable for subcutaneous tissue and nylon for skin, usually 2-0 or 3-0
- Surgical drains, e.g. Penrose
- Extraocular kit and fine suture material should entropion surgery also be necessary

are removed they will be much more comfortable and will see far better. Unfortunately, many owners are resistant to any surgery which alters the dog's face. Taking time to explain the procedure and its advantages to the owners will improve compliance and is something that nurses can do. Showing photographs of previous patients who have undergone the same procedure is also useful.

Brow sling procedure

Another method of correcting the heavy brow conformation, which retains the characteristic wrinkles, is the brow-lift or brow-sling procedure. With this procedure, several strips of braided polyester mesh are threaded though skin incisions from approximately 5 cm dorsal to the orbital rim down to the eyelid margin, and back up again where they are tightened and secured to lift the wrinkles. The mesh is then anchored to the periosteum to prevent slippage. Thus, the wrinkles are basically moved dorsally away from the eyelid margin. By anchoring them to the dorsal periosteum, a firm adhesion should be maintained. The small skin incisions are then closed. Owner compliance with this procedure is usually good, but it can have complications. Skin infections are frequently present within the skin folds of these dogs and need to be fully controlled prior to surgery. Sometimes infection can track along the polyester mesh, and fistulae can develop. The periosteal attachments can also break down due to the heavy weight of the skin, resulting in slippage and recurrence of the ocular signs.

Stades procedure

One final procedure for correcting upper lid entropion due to a 'slipped facial mask' (as seen in the cocker spaniel most commonly; see Fig. 7.4, p. 106), is the forced-granulation tissue or Stades procedure. With this technique, a strip of tissue is removed from the upper lid, making the eye-side incision as close as possible to the eyelid margin. An ellipse of tissue is removed, and instead of suturing the open edges together the upper incision is sutured to the raw subcutis, about 2 mm from the lid incision. This leaves a strip of open wound which heals by secondary intention. By doing so, a smooth scar develops in which no hair follicles are present and the trichiasis is thus corrected. Obviously, the owner must be fully aware of the fact that the dog will have open wounds above its eyes! As with all eyelid surgery, no dermatitis must be present preoperatively. Sometimes the procedure needs combining with a face-lift (rhytidectomy).

Medial canthal surgery

Surgery at the medial canthus requires magnification with an operating microscope. The two most common procedures performed in this region are the medial canthoplasty and repair of nasolacrimal duct lacerations. A medial canthoplasty shortens the palpebral fissure and is usually performed in brachycephalic patients. Care must be taken to avoid inadvertent damage to the nasolacrimal punctae, especially the ventral one through which the majority of tears drain. In addition to an extraocular kit, the surgeon might require some large suture material (e.g. 2-0 nylon) to thread into the nasolacrimal punctae so that their location is easily marked. The surgeon removes small pieces of eyelid tissue from upper and lower lids, and usually the caruncle is also removed. The wounds are sutured with 6-0 absorbable suture, usually in a double layer. This procedure is useful for dogs with epiphora and the combination of medial entropion, hairs on the caruncle and poor nasolacrimal drainage (see p. 113).

Lacerations of the medial eyelid region can involve damage to the nasolacrimal punctae or duct. If lacerated, the duct must be accurately sutured using fine absorbable material, such as 8-0 to 10-0 polygalactin 910. A cannula or piece of suture material will be left in the duct for a couple of weeks after surgery to ensure that healing does not occlude the duct. The cannula or suture will be sutured to the skin ventral to the lower lid— butterfly tapes make this easier. Postoperative nursing involves keeping the area clean with gentle bathing and applying topical antibiotic drops. Systemic antibiotics and NSAIDs are usually required following nasolacrimal duct procedures, and it is normal for the patient to wear an Elizabethan collar for several days.

PAROTID DUCT TRANSPOSITION

Parotid duct transposition is a procedure performed to alleviate severe keratoconjunctivitis sicca. It is undertaken in cases which are not responsive to topical ciclosporin, where the only other alternative is very frequent topical lubricants (which are time consuming for the owner and often distressing for the patient). For the surgery, the main duct from the parotid salivary gland is dissected and re-routed to open into the conjunctival sac. The eye is then lubricated by saliva. The instruments and equipment required for this procedure are listed in Table 8.2. Before considering the procedure, it is vital to ensure that the patient can produce saliva properly. A drop of something bitter placed on the tongue (e.g. lemon juice or atropine drops) should make the animal produce saliva profusely. If this does not occur, it suggests that the patient does not produce enough saliva and, as such, parotid duct transposition surgery is unlikely to successfully treat the keratoconjunctivitis sicca. Atropine is not routinely used in the premedication of patients for parotid duct transposition since its action of drying secretions makes cannulation of the parotid duct much more difficult. Two methods of surgery are used: a closed approach where the procedure is performed via the mouth, and the more common open procedure which is discussed here.

Once the animal is anaesthetised, the fur is clipped from the cheek, extending from the lip up to the lower lid and from the nose to level with the ear in a large square. Initial skin preparation is undertaken, and then the surgeon will cannulate the parotid duct. The mouth is kept open with a gag and the nurse can assist to pull the lips back. The duct is located approximately 1 cm above the carnassial tooth, usually on a small papilla. It helps if the suture material used for cannulation is coloured rather than transparent, since the duct will be easier to identify and dissect. The suture is passed as far up the duct as possible and cut to leave 1 cm protruding from the opening. Some surgeons anchor this via a separate suture loop in the adjacent mucosa. The surrounding area is gently cleansed, and then the final skin prep performed, including flushing the conjunctival sac. Care must be taken to prevent dislodging the suture during this final preparation. The patient is moved into theatre.

The surgeon will usually wear magnifying loupes for the operation. A skin incision is made over the cheek and the tissue gently dissected to reveal the duct. The facial nerve and vein are identified and moved aside if necessary. The duct is dissected free and followed back to the salivary gland, and forwards toward the mouth. It is freed from the gum (some surgeons use a biopsy punch to do this). At this stage the surgeon will often ask the nurse to remind them to suture the oral defect at the completion of surgery! The instruments which have penetrated the oral cavity are not used again. The surgeon checks that the freed duct is long enough to reach the eye without being stretched and that it is not twisted. Blunt dissection to the conjunctival sac is undertaken, and a scalpel blade incises the conjunctiva. The duct is directed up through the subcutaneous tunnel. Several sutures (6–8) are used to anchor the papilla to the conjunctiva in the lateral fornix. It might be necessary to trim the papilla to get a neat fit. The suture guide cannulating the duct is then removed. The skin is closed routinely, and the nurse reminds the surgeon to close the oral wound!

Postoperative care involves preventing self trauma with the use of an Elizabethan collar. Systemic antibiotic and NSAIDS are given together with topical antibiotics and sometimes lubricants. Gentle massage over the cheek can be performed several times a day and after eating to promote saliva flow. The patient should be observed eating to check that the eye becomes moist. This can be

---

Table 8.2 List of equipment required for parotid duct transposition

- Magnification—surgical loupes
- Material for cannulating duct—monofilament nylon 2-0 to 0-0
- Mouth gag
- Fine forceps to assist cannulation of duct
- Vacuum cushion
- Surgical drapes
- General soft tissue surgical kit
- Extraocular kit
- Standard scalpel blade (No. 15)
- Sterile swabs (small ophthalmic size)
- 6-0 and 4-0 polyglactin 910
- 3-0 nylon

further tested using lemon juice on the tongue to stimulate salivation. Patients are normally hospitalised for 24 hours after surgery or until the surgeon is happy that the procedure has been successful.

Although the procedure is very successful it is not without long-term complications, and owners must be made aware of these. The most common problems are overproduction of saliva and salt deposition. The amount of saliva reaching the eye cannot be regulated and in some dogs can be excessive, especially in drooling types such as boxers and bulldogs. The overflow can lead to a facial dermatitis. The use of a barrier cream can help prevent soreness. In severe cases, the parotid duct can be partially ligated to reduce the flow. Salt deposits occur due to the higher mineral content of saliva compared to tears. The eyelids can become dry and crusted, and deposits on the cornea can be irritating. Changing the diet and using calcium-chelating drops can reduce this problem, but in some patients it is necessary to resort to superficial keratectomy. Occasionally, the duct can become blocked, requiring surgery to remove the blockage. If this is required, a cannula can be left in place for 2–4 weeks and regular massage continued to try to prevent further problems from developing.

CORNEAL SURGERY

Surgery to the cornea is commonly necessary in ophthalmic practice. Deep corneal ulcers, sequestra in cats, corneal lacerations and foreign bodies are all encountered. Further details of these conditions are discussed in Chapter 7—here we will only deal with the surgical techniques and nursing assistance required. We will consider the superficial keratectomy, conjunctival grafts, corneoscleral transposition, porcine small intestinal submucosa (SIS) grafts, tissue glue, corneal transplants, foreign body removal and treatment for lacerations. Nursing care is similar in each case and will be discussed at the end of this section.

Superficial keratectomy

A superficial keratectomy entails surgical removal of the anterior layers of the cornea, usually the

Table 8.3 Items required for superficial keratectomy

- Operating microscope and surgeon's chair
- Intraocular kit
- Surgical drapes
- Fixed-depth keratome (disposable) or Beaver blade
- BSS or other irrigating fluid
- Cellulose spears
- Contact lens if required postoperatively

epithelium and anterior stroma. General anaesthesia and magnification via an operating microscope are necessary. It is performed for non-healing superficial ulcers, sequestrum removal in cats, chronic bullous ulceration in cases of corneal endothelial degeneration with corneal oedema and recurrent ulceration. The extent of the surgery will obviously depend upon the size of the damaged area, and will vary from a small 2 mm square of tissue to the whole corneal surface. The use of a fixed-depth keratome is more accurate than free-hand surgery with a plain Beaver blade. The equipment required for this surgery is listed in Table 8.3.

Following superficial keratectomy, a bandage contact lens can be placed to promote ocular comfort and protect the delicate epithelial cells as they grow over the surgical site. Accurate measurement of the cornea is advised to ensure a good fit of the contact lens so that it is not lost early. A suture placed at the lateral canthus to partially close the eyelids can improve lens retention times. Healing is normally expected in 1–2 weeks.

Conjunctival graft

Conjunctival grafts are performed following superficial keratectomy if more than $1/3$–$1/2$ stromal depth has been removed. They provide physical support to the weakened cornea as well as bringing a direct supply of blood vessels and lymphatics which offer antibacterial and anticollagenase activity. Several different types of graft can be used, but the most common technique is the pedicle graft. Here a strip of conjunctiva is dissected from the bulbar conjunctiva parallel to the limbus and is rotated over the cornea and sutured directly

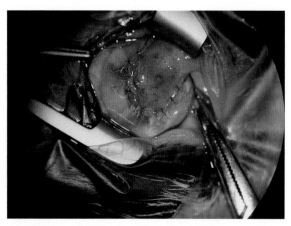

Fig. 8.2 Intraoperative appearance of a pedicle conjunctival graft. Note the sticky drape to prevent hair contamination and the use of mosquito forceps to stabilise the globe.

to the edges of the damaged tissue (Fig. 8.2). The pedicle should be large enough so that no tension is placed on it. It is harvested from the bulbar conjunctiva so that it moves with the eyeball and thus is not subjected to shearing forces. Normally, it is harvested from the dorsal conjunctiva but can come from any section. However, if the graft is perpendicular to the lids it is less likely to be rubbed and pulled off during blinking. The equipment needed for performing this surgery is the same as for a superficial keratectomy but with the addition of suture material. Normally, absorbable sutures are used, such as Vicryl, and sizes of 8–0 to 10–0 are chosen.

Once the cornea has fully healed following conjunctival grafting, a decision is made whether to trim the graft. This is performed under topical anaesthesia in most cases, and a fine pair of scissors (e.g. Steven's tenotomy scissors) are used to cut through the stalk of the pedicle. The remaining island of conjunctiva on the cornea is left to scar down and over the following weeks fades to a pale pink flat plaque. Sometimes the blood supply is left intact—for example, following the removal of a corneal sequestrum in a cat, as leaving the blood supply can help to prevent recurrence of the sequestrum. A balance has to be met between providing the best visual outcome by reducing the scarring as much as possible, countered with continued protection for the diseased cornea.

Corneoscleral transposition

Corneoscleral transposition is used to treat deep ulcers and sequestra in the visual axis. It is not recommended as a treatment for melting corneal ulcers. This is because the transposed cornea does not contain significant anti-collagenase activity (unlike the conjunctiva which is used for conjunctival grafts). As a result of this lack of anti-collagenase activity, the melting within the diseased cornea can spread to the newly grafted section of cornea, resulting in disease progression. This procedure has the advantage over conjunctival grafts of providing support via clear cornea. However, the surgery is technically more difficult and time-consuming. Under general anaesthesia, a superficial keratectomy is performed first, and then an advancement graft of cornea is created by dissecting a strip of cornea back to the limbus of approximately half stromal thickness. This strip is extended through the limbus and back into the conjunctiva over the sclera. Cautery might be required as the limbus dissection is made. The whole strip is then gently pulled forward and sutured into the keratectomy site. The only additional items required to perform this surgery to those for a superficial keratectomy are the suture material and microcautery unit. The end result is similar to a conjunctival graft except that the conjunctiva only reaches the edge of the keratectomy site, and this is filled with the transposed cornea instead.

Porcine small intestinal submucosa (SIS)

A recently introduced alternative to both conjunctival grafts and corneoscleral transposition surgery is the use of porcine small intestinal submucosa (SIS). This is a natural material which provides a scaffold for repair while providing physical support. It is collagen-based and comes in ready sterilised corneal discs which are trimmed to size and rehydrated in balanced salt solution (BSS) prior to suturing into the keratectomy site. Less scarring is reported compared to conjunc-tival grafts. Although they have been used for sequestra in cats, some reformation of the sequestra has occurred. Thus, they are usually recommended for deep ulcers and occasionally full thickness defects, although for the latter a supporting conjunctival pedicle graft might also be required. They are not recommended for melting ulcers.

Tissue glue

Tissue glues are used to treat small but deep ulcers and occasionally perforations (although most ophthalmologists do not recommend using glue if the cornea has perforated). Some people also advocate their use for superficial ulcers. Cyanoacrylate adhesive (Histoacryl, B Braun, Germany) provides mechanical support and acts as a barrier to neutrophil migration, as well as possessing some weak antibacterial activity. Accurate placement of the glue is required to prevent early sloughing, and general anaesthesia and an operating microscope are advised. However, some ophthalmologists who are experienced with this treatment use it in conscious patients, providing they are cooperative! The surgical site is debrided and thoroughly dried before the glue is 'painted' on using a 27 gauge needle on a 1 ml syringe (Fig. 8.3). The cornea is carefully flushed with BSS. Healing is complete within weeks, and the glue can be left to slough off naturally or can be removed with fine-toothed forceps under topical anaesthesia.

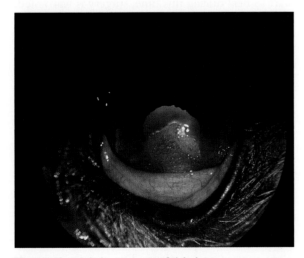

Fig. 8.3 Corneal glue on a superficial ulcer.

Corneal transplants

Corneal transplants are technically demanding procedures but offer the potential for a clear visual axis and are used for large deep ulcers and blinding endothelial disease. Homologous grafts are harvested from the same species, and although fresh donor grafts are preferred (as in human surgery) in veterinary ophthalmology we often resort to frozen grafts since these are more readily available. However, they are more likely to result in permanent scarring than fresh donor tissue. All tissue must be thoroughly defrosted before surgical use. The surgery is performed under general anaesthesia with neuromuscular blockade. Transplants can be partial thickness (lamellar) or full thickness (penetrating). Lamellar transplants are easier to perform since the recipient globe remains formed during the procedure and the globe is not actually entered—as such, postoperative uveitis is less severe. However, if the recipient corneal endothelium is damaged, this surgery will not result in any ocular clearing and, as such, a full thickness transplant is necessary.

A corneal trephine is used to harvest the donor tissue and must be 1–2 mm larger than the recipient site. For full thickness transplants, the recipient needs to have the globe supported during the surgery since a large area of cornea is to be removed. This is achieved by suturing a metal supporting ring to the limbus using 6-0 silk or Vicryl sutures. A corneal trephine is used to delineate the area to be removed, but it is not allowed to penetrate the cornea fully. Instead, a stab incision is made and the button of cornea is removed with corneal scissors following the demarcation of the trephine. The cornea is not fully removed by the trephine, as this could damage the delicate corneal endothelium surrounding the area to be removed. Viscoelastic material is injected into the anterior chamber, and the donor cornea is placed into the defect and sutured in place with simple interrupted 8-0 to 10-0 nylon sutures. The viscoelastic is flushed out with BSS before the final suture is placed.

Once the surgery is complete, postoperative treatment aims to prevent graft rejection. Thus, high levels of anti-inflammatory agents are used both topically and systemically. A typical protocol could include topical corticosteroids and ciclosporin, plus systemic NSAIDs and both topical and systemic antibiotics. Topical atropine can be used if extensive uveitis presents. Immediate complications include leaking from the wound, hyphaema and severe uveitis (which can include chorioretinitis and retinal detachments) and endophthalmitis. Later complications include graft rejection, corneal oedema and opacification of the donor tissue.

Thermal keratoplasty

A recently introduced surgery for the treatment of chronic corneal ulceration (bullous keratopathy) secondary to corneal endothelial degeneration is thermal keratoplasty. This should only be considered in eyes which are blind or severely visually impaired, with recurrent painful ulcers which cannot be managed by conventional means. It is salvage surgery for the eye. Under general anaesthesia, a blunt-tipped handheld cautery unit is used to make small burns into the corneal stroma, often 200–400 per eye. The procedure is best performed with the use of an operating microscope for accurate burn placement. A contact lens can be placed to promote ocular comfort postoperatively. The burns cause significant scarring, and this acts as a barrier to further bullous formation and thus prevents further ulceration. However, the scarring is often excessive, rendering the potential for vision minimal. Careful client education is required prior to considering this procedure.

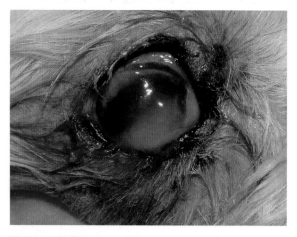

Fig. 8.4 Melting corneal ulcer (complication following routine cataract surgery).

The melting ulcer

The melting ulcer is both a medical and often a surgical emergency (Fig. 8.4). Without accurate diagnosis and appropriate treatment, the eye could well be lost. Melting ulcers can be seen in all species and are a potential complication from any ulcer. They can also develop following the use of topical steroids. They are characterised by a rapidly progressing liquefaction (melting) of the corneal stroma caused by excessive protease and collagenase activity. This melting activity can come from exogenous sources, such as *Pseudomonas* bacteria, or from excessive action of endogenous fibroblasts and white blood cells.

Swift recognition of the problem and aggressive treatment are needed to prevent corneal rupture and the need for enucleation. The usual approach to treatment includes the use of frequent topical antibiotics (based on Gram-staining initially, although swabs should be taken for both bacterial and fungal culture and sensitivity). Fortified solutions can be used. Topical atropine and sometimes NSAIDs are also employed. Topical anti-collagenase agents, such as EDTA or autologous serum, can help. For the latter, blood is drawn from the patient, spun down, and the serum then applied topically on an hourly basis. If stored in the fridge, the serum can be kept for a couple of days before being replaced with fresh supplies. The patient is hospitalised and medicated around the clock for 24–48 hours. If the cornea does not stabilise and start to heal during this time, surgery is warranted. This will entail removal of all unhealthy corneal stroma and the placement of a conjunctival pedicle graft. Usually, the frequency of topical medication can then be reduced to 4–6 times daily, and the patient can be discharged 1–2 days postoperatively, providing the owner is able to medicate easily. The prognosis must be guarded, but in some cases the eye can be salvaged and reasonable vision maintained.

Foreign body removal

Corneal foreign bodies are frequently encountered in ophthalmic practice. They are usually plant matter or cat claws. The severity depends

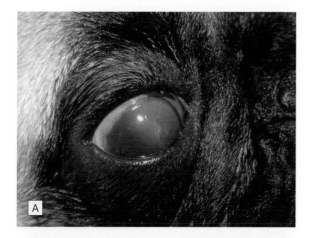

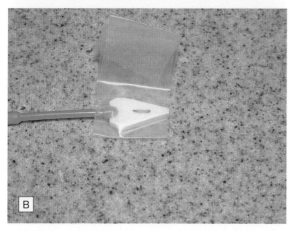

Fig. 8.5 a) superficial corneal foreign body in a Boston terrier b) small thorn removed.

very much on the type of material and the depth of penetration. Superficial objects can often be flushed out or gently removed with a sterile surgical spear (Fig. 8.5). However, items which are embedded within the cornea, perforated through it, or impaled within the lens or iris tissue require precise microsurgical removal (Fig. 8.6). The surgeon should be able to deal with any potential complications prior to attempting removal. If the surgeon is not able to suture the cornea or retrieve fragments of material from the anterior chamber, the case should be referred to someone who can. The nurse should be prepared for any complications and have corneal suture material ready, together with viscoelastics and so on in addition to the surgical kits should intraocular surgery prove necessary.

Many objects can be removed via the entry site by using a fine needle or foreign body spud to gently fix the material perpendicular to its long axis and gently rotate it out from the cornea (Fig. 8.7). The foreign body should never be grasped with forceps since this is likely to force the object deeper into the cornea. If the object has penetrated through the cornea and impaled on the lens or iris tissue, removal needs to be via a limbal incision. The eye is filled with viscoelastic to keep its shape and protect the endothelium

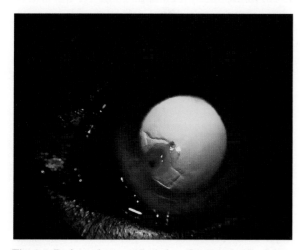

Fig. 8.6 Perforated corneal body in a German shepherd dog.

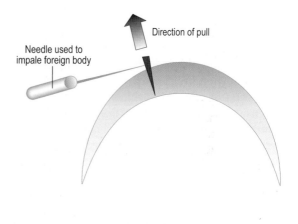

Direction of pull

Needle used to impale foreign body

Fig. 8.7 Removal of a corneal foreign body.

while intraocular forceps are used to gently remove the foreign body and any fragments. The corneal defects are sutured as necessary. Once the foreign body has been removed, the eye is treated with topical antibiotics, atropine and sometimes NSAID drops, although often these are given systemically. Providing the lens has not been badly damaged, the prognosis should be good. Injuries which do involve severe lens damage are discussed below.

Corneal laceration

Superficial corneal lacerations do not require specialist attention and can be treated as a shallow ulcer. However, deeper injuries, especially if obliquely though the cornea or jagged and irregular, should be repaired surgically. Any devitalised tissue is debrided, although this should be kept to a minimum to prevent distortion of the cornea. Direct sutures should be placed using 8-0 to 10-0 polygalactin 910 (Vicryl, Ethicon) or nylon. If the laceration has extended over the limbus and into the sclera, the prognosis is less good—more uveitis and hyphaema will be present as a result of damage to the underlying ciliary body. These can lead to blinding complications. In addition, ruptures in the sclera will weaken the structural support of the globe, and panophthalmitis can develop due to the introduction of pathogenic material into the posterior segment.

Iris prolapse

Prolapse of the iris through a corneal rupture can occur following progression of a corneal ulcer to perforation or after a full-thickness laceration. As soon as the cornea is perforated, aqueous will leak from the hole and the anterior chamber will start to collapse. The iris moves forwards to plug the gap, and some iris tissue usually protrudes though the cornea (Fig. 8.8a). It will appear dark and shiny if acutely presented, but with time it may dry out and occasionally can be confused for a foreign body. However, careful assessment of the eye will reveal a misshapen pupil, reduced depth of the anterior chamber, and often blood-stained

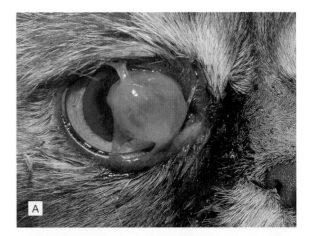

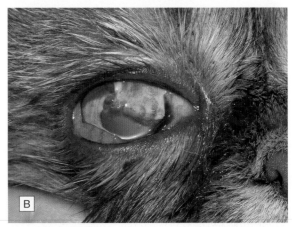

Fig. 8.8 Iris prolapse: a) in a cat following a cat-fight and corneal laceration; b) same eye post-surgery with conjunctival graft.

fibrin in the anterior chamber. The eye will also be very soft on gentle digital palpation.

Any iris prolapse should be treated as an emergency, and rapid surgical repair will offer the best prognosis. The general approach is to replace all viable iridal tissue and resect any that is devitalised. Surgery should be performed within 8 hours of the prolapse to offer the best prognosis. A general intraocular kit is necessary together with iris repositors, viscoelastic material, as well as BSS and microcautery to cut any devitalised tissue away. If cautery is not available, the iris can be cut with fine sharp scissors but bleeding is more likely to occur. Once all healthy tissue has been replaced and the anterior chamber filled, the corneal defect must be repaired. For laceration this can be achieved by direct suturing, but if a ruptured ulcer is present a conjunctival graft might be necessary (Fig. 8.8b).

Postoperatively, it is necessary to control the inevitable uveitis. Topical steroids might be required even though the cornea is compromised. If they are used, the patient should be hospitalised and regularly monitored for signs of corneal ulceration or melting. Uncontrolled uveitis can lead to synechia formation and secondary glaucoma. Another main complication is infection. Pathogenic organisms could have been introduced to the anterior chamber, and a panophthalmitis could develop. Thus, carefully chosen topical antibiotics are mandatory.

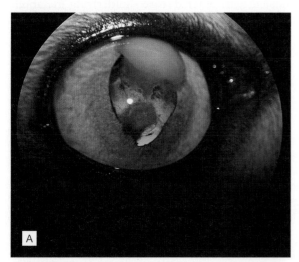

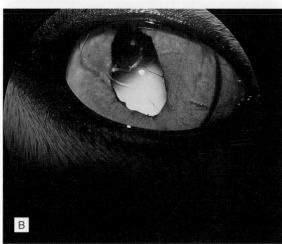

Fig. 8.9 Corneal laceration with lens involvement: a) the white material in the anterior chamber is lens cortex; b) same eye following phacoemulsification of the lens.

Lens assessment with corneal injuries

With any corneal laceration or iris prolapse, it is essential that full evaluation of the lens is undertaken. Any damage must be assessed and treated appropriately. Cat claw lacerations often appear to only involve a tear in the cornea, but the lens could also have been perforated. The anterior lens capsule must be carefully checked. Any leakage of lens material into the anterior chamber can result in a very serious uveitis—sometimes not developing immediately but after a delay of 1–2 weeks. In these cases, the corneal injury is repaired, and the patient appears to be doing well. Suddenly, an uncontrollable uveitis develops, leading to secondary glaucoma and eventual enucleation. If the lens is damaged, it is often preferable to remove it via phacoemulsification at the same time as repairing the cornea (Figs 8.9a & b). A uveitis will still develop, but it is more likely to respond to medication and vision is likely to be maintained. This will also prevent the development of a cataract which can occur following trauma. Clearly, lens involvement is a much more serious injury, and the owners should be fully aware that the prognosis is therefore worse than with a simple corneal injury. However, with careful management and diligent medication, these challenging cases can do surprisingly well on occasion.

Nursing care for corneal surgery

For all the procedures described above the same nursing principles apply. Medical nursing will be necessary prior to surgery—this can range from just a few applications of antibiotic and atropine prior to emergency repair of an iris prolapse to several days of multiple frequent drops for a melting corneal ulcer. Once surgery has been scheduled, the theatre nurse will prepare the necessary instrumentation and check with the surgeon whether any extra items, such as microcautery or viscoelastic material, might be required. The nurse will attend to the surgeon during the procedure and assist on recovery. Postoperative medication is invariably required. For example, this can be simply 5 days of topical antibiotic drops following a routine superficial keratectomy, or might be much more complex, as is necessary following iris prolapse repair. Hospitalisation records need updating and discharge sheets preparing as necessary. The nurse can also liaise with the owners regarding how the patient is doing and when it is likely to be allowed home.

LENS

Cataract surgery

Patient assessment for surgery

Cataract surgery is the most commonly performed intraocular procedure in ophthalmic practice. Although it is routine surgery in many specialist clinics, it is not something to be undertaken lightly and there are many things to consider. It is elective surgery, meaning that it is not essential to the animal's welfare but is something that we chose to subject them to. The aim of surgery is to improve or restore vision such that quality of life is made as good as possible. Thus, the first thing we need to consider is whether the patient is likely to benefit from the procedure. Many dogs and some cats go blind through cataract formation, and their lifestyles might not be affected by this. Often dogs will still happily play with toys and run off the lead in parks despite not seeing. Their other senses (smell and hearing) take over, and certainly in familiar environments they function almost totally normally. However, other patients are severely disabled by their reduced vision. They can become withdrawn and disinterested in life, unwilling to go for walks or interact with other pets and sometimes become very nervous. In such cases, surgery is usually recommended.

Since many of our cataract patients are elderly, it is important to ensure that the change in their behaviour is solely due to vision loss and not connected with other disease—underlying metabolic problems such as uncontrolled diabetes mellitus or age-related cognitive function loss (i.e. senility). For example, it is always of concern if owners state that the dog is confused at home (e.g. staring at walls thinking that they are at the door) since animals blinded by cataracts do not usually do this. They do bump into furniture initially but usually learn their way around the home very quickly. Therefore, if they are not improving in this regard at home, it is sensible to consider alternative reasons for their apparent confusion.

Table 8.4 Ocular examination for cataract assessment

Examination test	Relevance
Pupillary light reflex (PLR)	A brisk direct and indirect (PLR) suggests good retinal function. However, a sluggish response can be due to other things (e.g. nervous dog) and the PLR can be unreliable—some dogs with advanced retinal degeneration will still retain a good PLR
Dazzle reflex	A good reflex suggests an intact pathway but the absence of a reflex is of concern
Schirmer tear test readings	Keratoconjunctivitis sicca can increase the risk of infection, slow healing and increase the risk of ulceration. It can also affect the choice of postoperative medication
Fluorescein test	Any ulcers must be treated and fully healed before surgery
Intraocular pressure	Low pressure can suggest uveitis which must be treated before surgery. Raised pressure (glaucoma) is often a contraindication for surgery
Gonioscopy	Examination of the drainage angle is essential in breeds at-risk from primary glaucoma
Electroretinography (ERG)	If there is any doubt about retinal function (e.g. poor PLR), if the retina cannot be directly visualised, and in PRA susceptible breeds an ERG should always be performed
Ocular ultrasound	Necessary to check for retinal detachment, vitreal liquefaction, presence of hyaloid vessels

Once we have established that the animal would potentially benefit from cataract surgery, we need to assess the suitability of the patient for this. A full ophthalmic examination is necessary to try to establish the cause for the cataracts and to ensure that no other ocular disease is present which could make the eye(s) unsuitable for surgery. The main things to consider are outlined in Table 8.4. In dogs, many cataracts are inherited, and these tend to follow a particular pattern of localisation within the lens and progression, depending on the breed. For example, the form of inherited cataract seen in the golden retriever starts at the posterior pole of the lens and can remain small with no affect on vision for many years. In some patients they never progress, but in a percentage they do and can result in blindness. Thus, the usual advice to owners of affected dogs is to have the animal checked on a 6-monthly basis and only to consider surgery should the cataract start to enlarge. The situation in the Staffordshire bull terrier is different. Here dogs as young as 6–12 months develop rapidly progressing cataracts and become blind in a very short period of time; these patients should have surgery sooner rather than later.

Age-related cataracts are probably the second most common form referred for surgery, and as our pet population is living longer, these are becoming more and more frequent. These eyes might have other ageing changes present, such as corneal oedema and retinal degeneration, and as such a thorough examination is necessary to check the suitability of the patient. Cataracts are also seen following uveitis and can cause lens-induced uveitis when they progress rapidly or become hyper-mature. These need careful assessment. If extensive adhesions are present within the eye, the surgery will be more difficult and the success rate lower. Any uveitis must be fully controlled prior to surgery. A further cause of cataracts which can be overlooked by general practitioners is retinal degeneration. Generalised progressive atrophy (GPRA) will cause secondary cataract formation and, as such, the lens opacity can be wrongly blamed for the loss of vision. If the retina cannot be examined, one must consider electroretinography to determine whether the retina is functional before embarking on any surgery.

Once the eyes have been fully assessed for the type of cataract and suitability for surgery we must look at the rest of the patient! A full clinical examination is required together with further diagnostic tests as listed in Table 8.5. Any concurrent disease must be stable (i.e. diabetes mellitus, cardiac insufficiency, atopy or other skin disease, etc.). If the patient is receiving medication for any condition, this must be evaluated since it can affect the choice of anaesthetic agents or post-operative treatment. Cataract surgery is not an emergency procedure, and it is important to do everything possible to make it as safe as possible, as well as improving the chances of a successful visual outcome. The temperament of the patient must also be considered. Aggressive dogs will be difficult to manage in the hospital and as out-patients for postoperative checks. If they need to

Table 8.5 Diagnostic tests required before cataract surgery

Test	Reason
Haematology and biochemistry panel	Check for metabolic disease which could affect anaesthetic and postoperative medication
Urine analysis	Check no renal insufficiency or diabetes mellitus
Blood pressure measurement	Hypertension could affect GA and postoperative treatment plan
Work-up for any concurrent disease, e.g. cardiac	Suitability for elective surgery and postoperative treatment plan
Diabetic patients need stability checked—fructosamine assay and glucose curves	Elective surgery can have a detrimental effect on unstable patients and large swings in glucose levels can increase postoperative uveitis

be muzzled and physically restrained each time a drop needs applying, this will put up their blood pressure and could affect intraocular pressure, weaken the suture line or cause intraocular bleeding—all of which could have disastrous consequences.

The owners must be able to medicate their pet. There is a lot of aftercare required on the part of the owners, and if they are physically unable to put the drops in as frequently as directed or return for the regular postoperative check-ups, the success of the operation could be compromised. They should be aware that a long-term commitment is needed. Once the initial postoperative period is over, they often still need to return for re-examinations 2 or 3 times a year to check for long-term complications, such as the development of glaucoma. They must also have realistic expectations regarding the surgery. The animal should regain good functional vision, such that it does not bump into things, can see a ball to play and is keen to interact normally again. Sometimes the patient will regain vision almost immediately, but in some animals it can take 2 or 3 weeks before a noticeable improvement is achieved. Expected success rates and potential complications need to be discussed.

In general, the short-term success rates with modern surgical techniques are very good (85–95%), but these reduce with time. The highest success rate is achieved in immature cataracts. The vision restored is not as good as before the cataracts developed—even with the implantation of an intraocular lens. These are placed routinely, and certainly patients with an artificial lens have better close vision than those without. Not all patients are suitable for the placement of an intraocular lens. If an intraocular lens is not placed and the patient remains aphakic, the patient will still see well but close vision is never very good. These animals usually continue to smell their way to titbits and so on, rather then being able to catch them mid-air! Although many owners do report that their pet has a 'new lease of life' once they can see again, the operation does not turn a 12-year-old into a puppy, and their pet might not want to chase the cat again even if he can see it (perhaps simply because he is older and wiser)! Owners must be realistic in this respect.

Potential complications of cataract surgery are numerous! They include excessive uveitis or corneal ulceration, which can lead to scarring such that vision is not as good as was hoped, to severe problems such as glaucoma or retinal detachment which can result in permanent blindness. Thankfully, these severe complications are quite uncommon, but they still need to be discussed with the owners.

Owners must also be fully appraised of the costs involved, both for the surgery and aftercare, and should any complications develop. In the UK, many of the patients referred for cataract surgery have insurance cover. Owners must check their insurance policy details carefully since these vary tremendously. Some companies will only cover for a year from the diagnosis of the cataract, and some will not cover congenital conditions. The level of cover can be relatively low, such that if the cataracts are secondary to diabetes mellitus, for example, the limit to cover could be reached very easily. Owners should be aware of these potential pitfalls with their insurance cover.

Once we have ascertained that the eyes are suitable, the patient is suitable and the owners are committed to the undertaking, only then can we proceed with surgery.

Preoperative procedures

Normally, all relevant tests, such as haematology and biochemistry, electroretinography and ultrasonography, will have been performed prior to admission for surgery. However, if any additional tests are required, these should be done as soon as possible. The patient is normally admitted to the hospital on the day before surgery—both to allow any extra tests to be performed and to start on the preoperative medication regime. Any medication (both for the eyes and for other problems) needs to be checked with the owner and referring veterinarian (if appropriate) and listed on the nursing record. The animal is allowed to settle into their cage—many owners will bring blankets or toys from home as a comfort. Details of hospitalising the blind patient are discussed in Chapter 4. The eye(s) require quite complicated medication prior to surgery, and a nursing chart should be provided with details of what is required and

Table 8.6 Topical medication in preparation for cataract surgery

Drug	Reason for application
Atropine	Dilate pupil and stabilise blood–aqueous barrier
Tropicamide (Mydriacyl, Alcon)	Dilate pupil
Phenylephrine	Dilate pupil
Topical steroid—prednisolone acetate or dexamethasone	Anti-inflammatory
Topical NSAID—keratolac (Acular, Allergan), dichlorphenac (Voltarol, Novartis), flurbiprofen (Ocufen, Allergan)	Anti-inflammatory and stabilise blood–aqueous barrier
Antibiotic, e.g. chloramphenicol	Reduce risk of infection

when. Details of the commonly used pre-surgical drops are given in Table 8.6. Protocols will vary according to surgeon preference. Normally, some medication is started the day before surgery, and then an intensive regime is begun 2 hours before the operation is scheduled.

The patient should have an intravenous catheter placed (often in the hind leg so that the anaesthetist has easy access during surgery) and receive its premedication as instructed. Many surgeons include an NSAID in the premed, although some prefer an intravenous dose of steroid at induction. The patient is anaesthetised and the eye(s) prepared for surgery routinely. Muscle-relaxant anaesthesia (neuromuscular blockade) is required and is detailed in Chapter 6.

Methods of cataract surgery

The preferred method of cataract extraction is by phacoemulsification. This involves making a small incision into the cornea (3.2 mm) and removing a piece of the anterior lens capsule (capsulorhexis). The surgeon might inject a coloured dye into the anterior chamber to help outline the anterior capsule and will always inject a viscoelastic material prior to capsulorhexis. The viscoelastic is a thick gel-like substance which has two main functions:

● to coat and protect the delicate corneal endothelium so that it is not damaged during the surgery
● to keep the anterior chamber formed so that the surgery can be more easily performed.

Further information on viscoelastic material is included in Chapter 2. Once a circular hole has been created in the anterior lens capsule the phacoemulsification handpiece is used to remove the lens (Fig. 8.10). The machine tip vibrates between 30 000–60 000 times per second, and this fragments the lens (similar to a jack-hammer breaking up the road surface). The handpiece has irrigation and aspiration ports which allow the broken pieces of lens to be removed from the eye. Once the lens is removed, the surgeon will switch to an irrigation–aspiration (I/A) handpiece. This has a

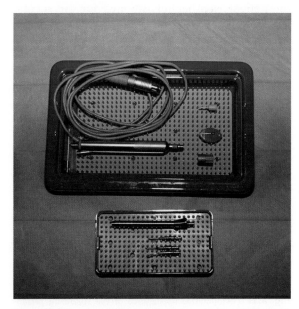

Fig. 8.10 Phacoemulsification handpiece (top) and I/A handpiece (bottom).

smaller rounded tip and can be used to gently remove any remaining lens fibres without the risk of damaging the delicate posterior lens capsule. This capsule is normally left intact (to keep the vitreous separate and reduce the risk of complications such as retinal detachment). However, if there is any opacity on the posterior capsule, the surgeon might decide to remove a section of it—usually just a small portion in the visual axis (i.e. the centre of the pupil). If a large piece of posterior lens capsule is removed, the surgeon might perform an anterior vitrectomy, for which the special vitrectomy handpiece will be needed. The I/A handpiece is used to 'vacuum' and 'polish' the remaining lens capsule.

If an intraocular lens is to be inserted, then further viscoelastic is placed in the eye to facilitate this. Some intraocular lenses require that the corneal incision is enlarged to allow them to be placed, but more recent designs fold up and can be injected through the same small incision. The lens is centred in the capsular bag, and any remaining viscoelastic material is removed (Fig. 8.11). Some surgeons inject a pupil-constricting agent into the eye at this stage, while others wait until the surgery is complete and place a drop topically. The corneal wound is sutured (with 8–0 to 10–0 polygalactin 910 or monofilament nylon), and the patient is either repositioned for the second

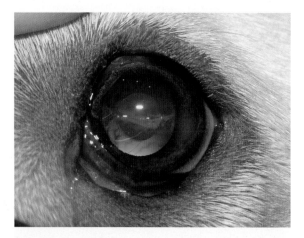

Fig. 8.11 Postoperative appearance of eye following phaco-emulsification and intraocular lens implantation (2 weeks post operation).

eye to undergo surgery or is allowed to recover from anaesthesia.

The second method for cataract surgery is now less common. The extracapsular technique involves making a large incision in the cornea close to the limbus—extending 150–180 degrees. A large piece of anterior lens capsule is removed, and the lens is scooped out whole. Any remaining pieces of lens material are flushed out, the cornea is sutured and the collapsed anterior chamber is reformed. This method is more traumatic to the eye and carries a lower success rate, mainly due to increased uveitis postoperatively.

A final method of lens extraction is the intracapsular technique—here the lens is removed with its capsule. It is only suitable for unstable (luxated or subluxated) lenses and is discussed later in the section on lens luxation.

The role of the nurse during cataract surgery

It is the role of the nurse to get all equipment ready for cataract surgery, together with all the instruments and ancillary items which will be required. These are listed in Table 8.7. The nurse will switch on the machines and do any calibration checks which might be required. All instrument kits must be checked for sterility. If the irrigating fluids are 'home made', these should be prepared and labelled. Although specific products are available, many veterinary ophthalmologists simply formulate their own—usually taking lactated Ringer's solution (Hartmann's) and adding a variety of agents to this. Heparin is added to reduce fibrin formation and reduce uveitis, adrenaline for haemostasis and to help maintain pupil dilation, and sodium bicarbonate to simulate the pH of aqueous and protect the corneal endothelium.

It is usual to have an anaesthetist; so the nurse should not need to worry about the anaesthesia at all and can concentrate on assisting the surgeon. Some surgeons prefer to have a scrubbed assistant as well during the procedure, although this is not always necessary. The theatre nurse will help to position the patient for surgery, but the exact positioning is left to the surgeon who will check this by looking down the microscope and adjusting the patient's head to ensure the best visualisation of

> **Table 8.7** Equipment and instruments required for cataract surgery
>
> - Operating microscope (and surgeon's stool)
> - Vacuum pillow
> - Phacoemulsification machine
> - Tubing for phacoemulsification machine (manifold set)
> - Intraocular irrigation fluid
> - Phacoemulsification handpiece and needle
> - Any other phacoemulsification disposables
> - I/A handpiece
> - Surgical drapes
> - Intraocular kit
> - Cataract kit
> - Cataract 'knife' or blade for incision
> - Blue colour cap dye
> - Viscoelastic material
> - Intraocular lens
> - Intraocular lens inserter and forceps
> - 23 gauge needle with insulin syringe (for capsulorhexis)
> - Cellulose spears (swabs)
> - Vitrectomy handpiece (optional)
> - Miotic agent—Miochol, carbachol or latanoprost drops
> - Suture material—nylon or polyglactin 910, 8-0 to 10-0

coemulsification machines enable the surgeon to adjust the power and vacuum settings, but often the nurse will be asked to change these if required. The nurse should also be prepared to fetch any extra items which the surgeon might request, such as a vitrectomy handpiece should it be necessary to remove some of the vitreous gel, or 1:10 000 adrenaline (epinephrine) should the pupil become constricted such that the surgeon cannot visualise the lens properly.

Once the surgery is completed and the patient starts to recover, the nurse can apply foot bandages if required and any topical medication—some ophthalmic surgeons favour a miotic (e.g. carbachol) or an anti-glaucoma drop, such as latanoprost (Xalatan, Pharmacia) or dorzolamide (Trusopt, MSD), at the end of surgery.

The instruments are cleaned and sterilised routinely. The phacoemulsification and I/A handpieces need to be flushed and cleaned according to the manufacturer's recommendations. The phacoemulsification machine itself might require flushing before being switched off and stored for future use. The protocols for this vary from machine to machine.

the eye. Patients are usually in lateral or dorsal recumbency—the latter makes it easier to move to the second eye during bilateral procedures. Vacuum pillows are essential for accurate and secure positioning. Once the patient is positioned and the microscope adjusted, it is essential that nothing is moved! Knocking against the table or the microscope can significantly impair the surgeon's visibility, and if instruments are in the eye at the time the consequences can be disastrous.

The surgeon scrubs, gowns and gloves, and then sits in position for the nurse to open the various sterile kits and disposables and set-up the phacoemulsification machine with the tubing and fluid lines. Most machines need tuning at this stage, and the surgeon will instruct as to which buttons to press! The nurse must monitor the fluid levels during surgery, and if these are getting low, must warn the surgeon who will stop operating while a fresh supply of irrigating fluid is connected. Low fluid pressure or air in the tubing can have deleterious effects within the eye. Some pha-

Postoperative care

The patient is allowed to recover from anaesthesia in a warm, quiet environment. The eyes must be closely monitored in the first few hours—the wound must not leak, no haemorrhage should develop and the cornea should remain clear. If there is any change in appearance of the eye or in the behaviour of the patient (e.g. suddenly wanting to rub or holding the eye closed), the surgeon must be informed immediately. Intraocular pressure is often checked several times in the 12–24 hours following surgery. Postoperative ocular hypertension is a complication which needs to be recognised and treated with urgency to avoid sight-threatening damage. Some ophthalmologists favour routine use of anti-glaucoma medication for this reason.

The patient is usually prescribed several topical medications following surgery. These include an antibiotic for 7–10 days (sometimes longer in diabetic patients), steroids (e.g. prednisolone acetate) to reduce inflammation, NSAIDs (e.g. keratolac) for the same reason and tropicamide to help keep the pupil moving. The mydriasis caused by tropicamide is short acting, and so the pupil constricts as it wears off—the movement helps to reduce synechia formation. Atropine is sometimes prescribed instead of tropicamide if moderate uveitis is present. In addition to opening the pupil, the atropine helps to stabilise the blood–aqueous barrier. Systemic medication usually includes a broad-spectrum antibiotic and NSAID, or occasionally a systemic steroid such as prednisolone.

Discharge instructions

Once the animal is ready to be returned to its owners (sometimes later on the day of surgery or sometimes after 2–3 days of hospitalisation), it is important for the nurse to go through the discharge instructions with the owners before bringing their pet out to them—as soon as they see their dog or cat again they will stop listening to what is being told! Written instructions should back up the verbal advice. If foot bandages are still present or the patient has an Elizabethan collar, instructions regarding how long these must be worn should be given. Owners should be clear about what medication needs to go into the eye and how frequently, and about leaving sufficient time between different topical agents (usually 10 minutes or longer). They should be aware that the patient must be kept very quiet for the coming days to weeks—no playing roughly, chasing toys, leaping up on the settee, barking at the postman and so on. If they have any questions which the nurse cannot answer (e.g. details about the surgical procedure), the nurse should make sure that the surgeon contacts the owner to answer specific queries. If the owner has any worries or concerns once they have taken their pet home, they should be instructed to contact the practice. An appointment should be made for the first recheck and only then should the patient be released back to the care of the owner.

Lens luxation

Surgery is often necessary for lens luxations. This condition is commonly seen as a primary (inherited) problem in several terrier breeds (see Table 7.10) and occasionally in the border collie and Shar-pei. It is a very serious disease which often results in blindness, even if managed correctly. Secondary lens luxation is more common in cats following chronic uveitis, but also occurs in dogs following uveitis although is more frequently associated with glaucoma and globe enlargement.

Lens luxation occurs when the lens fibres which hold it in position weaken and break, allowing the lens to slip and fall into the anterior or posterior segments. If it falls backwards, into the posterior segment, the lens can often be left in situ. Miotics, including anti-glaucoma medications such as latanoprost, can be used medically to reduce the risk of the lens falling forwards. However, urgent surgical removal is required if the lens rests in the anterior chamber (Fig. 8.12). If not removed within hours of an anterior luxation, the secondary glaucoma which develops can cause permanent blindness.

Intraocular pressure is measured prior to surgery and if elevated, which it often is, the patient might require a mannitol infusion. This is given once adequate renal function has been demonstrated. General anaesthesia for lendectomy is required, and neuromuscular blockade makes the surgery easier to perform. The patient is prepared for surgery routinely, and the equipment and instruments required are listed in Table 8.8.

The patient is positioned in theatre by the surgeon since the view down the microscope must be

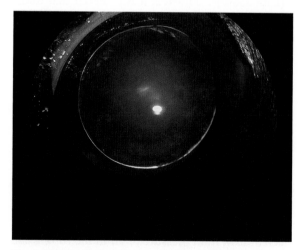

Fig. 8.12 Anterior lens luxation in a Tibetan terrier.

Table 8.8 Equipment and instruments required for lens luxation surgery

- Operating microscope (and surgeon's stool)
- Vacuum pillow
- Surgical drapes
- Intraocular kit
- Beaver blade for corneal incision
- Viscoelastic material
- Plain or irrigating vectis (with irrigating fluid if the latter)
- BSS (balanced salt solution) or other suitable irrigating fluid
- Cryoprobe and extraction unit if available
- Cellulose spears
- Vitrectomy handpiece and unit
- Intraocular lens for suture fixation (optional)
- Suture material—nylon or polyglactin 910

exactly right. The nurse opens the sterile kits as required and sets up any equipment or fetches extra items as required.

The surgery for lens luxation involves making a large incision in the cornea close to the limbus. Prior to this, a lateral canthotomy can be performed to assist access. The need for this varies according to the skull anatomy of the patient and whether muscle-relaxant anaesthesia is used (if it is not then a canthotomy is essential to get good surgical access). Viscoelastic material can be injected to protect intraocular structures. Removal of the entire lens is achieved with either a lens loop (vectis) to scoop the lens out, or a cryoprobe to adhere to the lens and then gently withdraw it. The lens should always be removed very slowly to ensure that no traction is placed on the ciliary body via remaining lens fibres (this would result in significant haemorrhage), and to make sure that no vitreous is pulled out with the lens (which could trigger glaucoma or a retinal detachment).

Once the lens is successfully removed the eye is flushed. If necessary, a partial vitrectomy can be performed. Some surgeons place intraocular lenses which are sutured into position, but these are not used as commonly as with cataract surgery. The corneal incision is closed with a continuous suture of 8–0 to 10–0 polyglactin 910 or nylon, depending on surgeon preference. The canthotomy incision is closed with 6-0 absorbable material. Some lens luxations are amenable to

removal by phacoemulsification—providing it is possible to stabilise the loose lens sufficiently to allow this. All the equipment listed for cataract surgery will be required if phacoemulsification is attempted. An advantage of this method is the small incision required and less disruption to intraocular contents. However, it runs the serious disadvantage of the loose lens falling into the posterior segment during the procedure, which can have catastrophic consequences.

Postoperative care for lens luxation surgery follows the same principles as cataract and other intraocular procedures. The patient must be kept quiet with minimal exercise and must be prevented from rubbing with suitable analgesia and an Elizabethan collar or foot bandages. Topical treatment usually consists of an antibiotic for 7–10 days, plus several weeks of anti-inflammatory drops (usually steroid-based) and often anti-glaucoma drops as well (e.g. dorzolamide, Trusopt MSD).

In addition to ensuring owner compliance regarding aftercare, it is important to explain what to expect in terms of vision following surgery. Lens luxation is an emergency, and pets go from having normal vision to blindness very quickly. Once the lens has been removed, even if glaucoma has not developed or has been fully controlled, vision is worse after surgery than it was before the pet developed the condition (Fig. 8.13). Owners often do not realise this and can be disappointed.

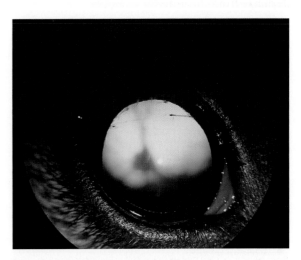

Fig. 8.13 Aphakic appearance of the eye 1 month post lendectomy—the lack of lens means that the optic disc can be clearly seen in the tapetal reflex.

If the time is taken to explain that it will take a short while for their pet to adapt to the change in their vision, and that the surgery aims to prevent the pain and permanent blindness caused by acute glaucoma, most owners accept that a comfortable pet with blurred vision is by far the best outcome, and their expectations are more realistic. Unfortunately, the long-term prognosis for maintaining vision remains guarded since glaucoma can develop 2–3 years after successful lendectomy. The owners must be aware that regular re-examinations and intraocular pressure checks will be required long-term—this is not a one-off operation to cure their pet!

GLAUCOMA SURGERY

The treatment of glaucoma is often specialised, and referral should always be considered. Unfortunately, many general practitioners do not have access to tonometry, and without being able to measure intraocular pressure it is impossible to accurately assess responses to treatment. The clinical signs, causes and medical management of glaucoma are discussed in Chapter 7, and in Tables 7.11–7.14. In this section, we will consider the specialised surgical techniques which can be undertaken. These rely on the same two principles as medical management—i.e. ways to reduce the production of aqueous humour and to improve its drainage from the anterior chamber.

Two surgical techniques are available to reduce the production of aqueous—cryosurgery (cyclo-cryotherapy) and laser surgery (cyclophotoablation). Both procedures are non invasive: the ciliary body is reached via the sclera and the eye does not need to be opened at all. The equipment required is listed in Table 8.9. Both are performed under general anaesthesia. The eye is surgically prepared and a pair of callipers are used to accurately measure the site for probe placement—this is normally on the sclera 5 mm from the limbus. The exact positioning is essential to ensure that the correct ciliary body cells are damaged by either the heat (laser) or extreme cold energy.

Cyclocryotherapy

Cyclocryotherapy is only used in blind eyes to reduce intraocular pressure to non-painful levels. It can induce shrinkage of the globe (phthisis bulbi), which is sometimes more cosmetic in appearance than a huge glaucomatous globe. Both liquid nitrogen and nitrous oxide can be employed successfully. The probe is usually 2–3 mm in diameter and is placed directly onto the bulbar conjunctiva in the correct site. Moderate pressure is applied for approximately 2 minutes. The probe is repositioned and the procedure repeated. In total, between 8–16 sites are frozen over the circumference of the globe, 5 mm posterior to the limbus, avoiding the 3 and 9 o'clock positions since the blood vessels which run through the sclera in this area are essential for ocular health.

Following cryosurgery there can be a significant rise in intraocular pressure. In many instances, paracentesis is required (removal of a small volume of aqueous) to relieve the pain associated with the sudden rise in pressure. It is common to do this once the surgery has been completed, but regular measurement of intraocular pressure over the following 12–24 hours is essential and further paracentesis might be required. Significant inflammation also follows cyclocryotherapy, and so topical and systemic anti-inflammatory agents are required for 2–3 weeks. Topical anti-glaucoma medication is also continued until stable, low levels of intraocular pressure are reached such that it can be carefully discontinued.

Table 8.9 Items required for laser or cryosurgery for glaucoma

- Cyclodestructive equipment—i.e. laser or cyro-unit with appropriate probes
- Callipers
- Eyelid speculum
- Rat-toothed forceps
- 2 pairs of mosquito forceps
- Suture material and needle holders for stay sutures (if used)
- Cellulose spears
- BSS and gallipot
- 1 ml syringe and 25 gauge needle for paracentesis

Cyclophotocoagulation

Cyclophotocoagulation causes less post-surgical inflammation and is less traumatic to the eye than cyclocryotherapy. It can be used in visual eyes or those with the potential for return of vision. Different types of laser are available, but the most commonly used type is the diode laser. Since lasers are generally effective only on pigmented tissue, laser surgery is not suitable in pale-eyed dogs (e.g. Siberian huskies). Health and safety issues must be addressed when lasers are employed—for example, safety goggles must be worn by all staff in the vicinity and a minimum number of people should be exposed to the potential hazards. The energy delivered and time per pulse of energy can be varied according to surgeon preference and the severity of glaucoma. In general, higher settings are used in end-stage permanently blind eyes. It is usual to apply the laser probe to between 30 and 40 sites around the circumference of the globe, avoiding the 3 and 9 o'clock positions as for cyclocryotherapy (Fig. 8.14). In the same way as pressure spikes occur following cryosurgery, they too can be expected following laser surgery, although they are often slightly less severe and do not continue for as long. Paracentesis might be required more than once in the few hours following the procedure.

Postoperative medication following laser surgery is similar to that for cryosurgery, with topical anti-inflammatory drops as well as continued anti-glaucoma medication. The post-surgical uveitis is usually less severe than with cryosurgery, and

eyes tend to be more comfortable. Possible complications (in addition to the pressure spikes) include corneal ulceration, intraocular haemorrhage, cataract formation and retinal detachment.

Anterior chamber drainage implants

The main surgical alternative to cyclodestructive procedures is the use of drainage implants. These have largely superseded previous surgical methods for improving aqueous outflow. They can be used in visual or potentially sighted eyes. Since the surgery is invasive and expensive, and attentive after care is required, it is not commonly performed in irreparably blind eyes. Various types of implant are available, but all consist of a small silicone tube which is inserted into the anterior chamber attached to a 'footplate' which is sutured to the sclera under the extraocular muscles. Aqueous drains out of the tube and collects around the footplate (a small bleb of fluid can be seen around the footplate). It then diffuses away into the surrounding tissues. Unfortunately, in dogs, scarring forms quickly around the footplate of the implant and prevents the bleb from forming such that

---

Table 8.10 Items required for anterior chamber shunt placement

- Operating microscope (and surgeon's stool)
- Intraocular kit
- Drapes
- BSS (balanced salt solution) or other irrigating fluid
- Cautery (for scleral bleeding)
- Cellulose spears
- Muscle hooks (to part extraocular muscles)
- Anterior chamber implant
- 20–22 gauge needle (to penetrate anterior chamber)
- Viscoelastic (to protect corneal endothelium during tube implantation and maintain a formed anterior chamber)
- Sutures
    - non-absorbable 7-0 to 9-0, to anchor implant to sclera
    - absorbable 6-0 to 8-0, to close conjunctival flap over implant
- Anti-metabolite, e.g. Mitomycin C to impede fibrosis around implant
- tPA (tissue plasminogen activator) to inject into anterior chamber to reduce fibrin production

---

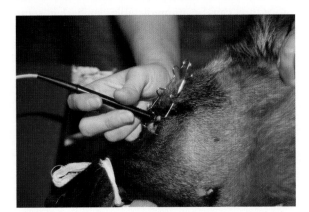

Fig. 8.14 Cyclophotocoagulation—laser handpiece placed on sclera.

aqueous cannot drain away and the pressure rises again. To try to prevent this, or at least slow the reaction such that the implant remains functional for longer, the use of anti-fibrotic agents is suggested. Anti-metabolites such as mitomycin-C are applied to the sclera where the implant is to be placed using a cellulose spear. It is important that the area is flushed with copious amounts of BSS or similar, and that the mitomycin-C does not touch the conjunctiva or enter the anterior chamber since it will prevent healing and cause a serious uveitis. The items required for implant surgery are listed in Table 8.10.

Following surgery, the intraocular pressure needs to be regularly checked. Some implants have one-way valves which prevent excessive drainage from the anterior chamber. If the pressure becomes very low (hypotony, below 5 mmHg), this can exacerbate uveitis and affect intraocular health. Patients will receive intensive anti-inflammatory medication (both topically and systemically), together with continued anti-glaucoma drops if required.

Although drainage implants are fairly successful, patients need close monitoring since there are several serious complications which can occur. In addition to fibrosis around the footplate preventing drainage, a more immediate complication of fibrin blocking the drainage tube is quite common. In this case, the bleb of aqueous collecting around the footplate will flatten and aqueous flare and fibrin will be seen in the anterior chamber. Intraocular pressure will rise quickly. The drainage tube will need to be flushed with further tPA (tissue plasminogen activator) to break down the fibrin clots. This obviously requires another general anaesthetic. Other complications include serious ongoing uveitis which further exacerbates the glaucoma, damage to the iris or cornea due to inaccurate tube placement, extrusion of the footplate or tube from the anterior chamber and continued reduction in the normal outflow facility such that the drainage tube is unable to divert sufficient aqueous to keep the pressure controlled. Severe panophthalmitis and infections can also occur on rare occasions such that enucleation is required.

Other surgical drainage procedures

The use of anterior chamber shunts has largely replaced the previous techniques to improve aqueous drainage in glaucomatous eyes. Unfortunately, they all have complicated names—iridencleisis, cyclodialysis and scleral trephination are each performed occasionally. Iridencleisis involves taking a piece of iris and suturing it to the subconjunctival space through a limbal incision. The aim is to allow aqueous to flow out into the subconjunctival space—the sutured iris acts like a wick to draw out the aqueous. With cyclodialysis, a fistula is created from the anterior chamber into the sclera and subconjunctival space beneath the iris and ciliary body. Trephination is similar with the creation of a hole at the limbus allowing aqueous to escape into the subconjunctival tissue. A piece of peripheral iris must be removed to prevent this from plugging the hole. Each of these procedures only lasts for a few months before the new drainage channels scar and close over, and as such they are now rarely undertaken.

Procedures for blind, end-stage glaucoma

Animals which are permanently blind and in pain from raised intraocular pressure need to have some form of treatment for humane reasons. Enucleation is commonly performed and is discussed in Chapter 7. Two other alternatives to this are intravitreal genticin injections and the use of intrascleral prosthesis. The former involves injecting a calculated dose of genticin (sometimes with steroid as well) into the posterior segment which is toxic to the ciliary body and destroys it. Eyes often become shrunken (phthisis bulbi) but are usually comfortable. However, the procedure can be unpredictable, such that some patients have minimal change in their intraocular pressure. Significant panuveitis is caused by the injection. However, the procedure can be performed in high-risk patients for which lengthy general anaesthesia and surgery are not recommended. It should not be performed in cats (due to the risk of triggering the development of post-traumatic intraocular sarcoma). Intrascleral prosthesis are discussed below in the section on the orbit.

SURGERY ON THE UVEAL TRACT

Surgical procedures on the uveal tract are not performed as commonly as corneal or lens surgery, or that for glaucoma. However, paracentesis is undertaken routinely to collect samples of aqueous. Repair of corneal lacerations involving prolapse of iris tissue was discussed above in the section on cornea. Surgery for iris cysts, iris neoplasia and iris bombe can all be carried out.

Paracentesis

Paracentesis is the collection of aqueous from the anterior chamber. It should be performed under general anaesthesia in most cases. It involves taking a fine gauge needle (e.g. insulin or tuberculin needle and syringe) to aspirate a small volume (0.1–0.3ml) of aqueous. This can be processed for cytology, culture (both bacterial and fungal), and for titres of specific pathogens (e.g. *Toxoplasma*). The eye is routinely prepped for surgery, and the nurse should gather the necessary instrumentation (listed in Table 8.11). Postoperatively, one or two doses of topical atropine and 3–5 days of antibiotics are usually necessary, but this will vary depending on the underlying disease.

Removal of iris cysts

Iris cysts are benign fluid-filled structures which do not normally require any treatment. However, if they are multiple or large in size, such that they occlude the pupil and reduce vision, they can be removed. This is performed under general anaesthesia using an operating microscope for magnification. A small corneal incision is made and the cysts float up and out of the anterior chamber. Viscoelastic material can be injected to flush the cysts out. Alternatively, a needle can be used to

Table 8.11 Items required for paracentesis
• Eyelid speculum
• Syringe and needle (e.g. insulin, tuberculin or 1 ml syringe and 25–27 gauge needle)
• Fine-toothed forceps (e.g. Von Graefe fixation forceps)
• Sterile cellulose spears
• Equipment for aqueous analysis—microscope slides, sterile containers, bacterial swabs, etc.

burst the cysts. More recently, lasers have been employed to rupture the cysts. Fragments of pigmented uveal tissue will remain if the cysts are burst. These can attach to the posterior cornea or anterior lens capsule but do not require any further intervention. Topical antibiotics and one drop of atropine are used postoperatively.

Surgical removal of iris neoplasms

Discrete masses on the anterior iris, such as uveal melanoma in dogs, can be removed by cutting away a sector of iris containing the mass (which should be submitted for histological analysis). Before considering any surgery, both ocular ultrasonography and gonioscopy should be routinely performed. For sector removal, a corneal incision is made at the limbus and the cornea reflected to expose the iris. Sharp scissors can be employed to cut the iris, but this results in extensive bleeding and so a hand-held microcautery unit is preferred. Occasionally, ciliary body masses can be removed in a similar way, with the addition of a cyclodialysis spatula to dissect between the sclera and ciliary body so that a sector of this can also be removed. Even more haemorrhage can be expected with this surgery, and the complications of hyphaema must be discussed with the owner (such as refractory uveitis, synechia formation and secondary glaucoma). Postoperative medication includes intensive anti-inflammatory drugs (both topically and systemically) since the inevitable uveitis must be controlled if the surgery is to be successful.

More recently, lasers have been employed to treat pigmented uveal tumours. Diode lasers are most commonly used, and the surgery has the advantage of being non-invasive—the laser energy is delivered through the cornea onto the pigmented mass. The mass will shrink, but some pigment will remain flat within the iris and the owners must be made aware that this will be the case. Less uveitis develops and the risk of complication is lower than with conventional excisional surgery, but unfortunately no material is harvested for histopathology and the exact laser protocol required can vary from patient to patient, such that in some cases the surgery needs to be repeated.

Iris bombé

Iris bombé is the 360 degree attachment of the iris to the anterior lens capsule via posterior synechia. It follows uveitis and results in blockage of aqueous flow from its formation in the posterior chamber through the pupil to the iridocorneal angle. This blockage results in a rapid secondary glaucoma. Medical management with intensive anti-inflammatory agents and pupil dilators is tried initially. If this is unsuccessful, surgery might be warranted. Surgery to release the adhesions can be performed early in the course of the disease, but once the inflammatory membranes have strongly adhered this is not successful. Instead, a sector of iris should be removed or a laser can be used to blast holes though the iris, allowing the free flow of aqueous. Unfortunately, these often close quickly with the ongoing uveitis exacerbating the situation. Thus, the prognosis for iris bombé must always be guarded.

tPA—tissue plasminogen activator

tPA is commonly used in ophthalmic specialty practice to dissolve blood clots and fibrin in the anterior chamber. Fibrin forms from fibrinogen which enters the eye during inflammatory processes and with haemorrhage. As its name implies, tPA activates plasminogen which triggers the formation of plasmin, and it is this compound which lyses fibrin (see Fig. 2.4, p. 25 and Chapter 2 for more information). Excessive fibrin in the eye not only affects optical clarity but exacerbates intraocular damage through the formation of adhesions (synechiae), traction bands which can lead to retinal detachment, and the development of secondary glaucoma.

tPA is available in variable doses (usually 20 mg, 50 mg or 100 mg vials), but only very low doses are required for ocular use, typically just 25 µg. The vials are reconstituted and diluted to 25 µg in 100 µL and can be frozen in aliquots ready for use. Under general anaesthesia, following routine ocular preparation, 25 µg are injected into the anterior chamber. Dissolving of the blood or fibrin clot can be expected in 15–30 minutes.

Vitrectomy, removal of some or all of the vitreous, can be performed during cataract or lens luxation surgery. It can also be undertaken in refractory posterior uveitis and panophthalmitis. Samples should always be sent for laboratory investigation in these cases. Vitreocentesis (the taking of vitreous aspirates for laboratory analysis) can also be undertaken, usually for suspected posterior segment infections.

Vitrectomy is most commonly performed via an automated handpiece attached to a standard phacoemulsification machine, although dedicated vitrectomy units are also available. In veterinary ophthalmology, the anterior approach is the most commonly used—via a corneal or limbal incision and during surgery for cataracts or luxated lenses, as mentioned above. It is indicated if any vitreous is present in the anterior chamber or pupil—if present it must be removed to reduce the risk of complications such as glaucoma. Manual vitrectomy can also be performed, using cellulose spears to which the vitreous adheres prior to cutting with fine scissors. This method is obviously less accurate than with an automated cutting handpiece. Posterior vitrectomy can be performed via the sclera 5–7 mm posterior to the limbus. The instrumentation and equipment required is extremely specialised and very few veterinary ophthalmologists have access to it. However, it can be undertaken in cases of recurrent equine uveitis, endophthalmitis and prior to retinal reattachment surgery.

Vitreocentesis is performed under general anaesthesia following pharmacological pupil dilation (e.g. with tropicamide). Routine surgical preparation is undertaken, and a 20–25 gauge needle attached to a 0.5 or 1.0 ml syringe is placed 5–7 mm behind the limbus. Care must be taken to avoid damage to the ciliary body, lens and retina. The exact positioning of the needle will vary according to the species and breed, and the quadrant of the globe through which the sample is being taken. Using an indirect ophthalmoscope through the dilated pupil, the surgeon can visualise the needle tip and thus direct it to the area of vitreous which needs sampling. An equal volume of fluid should be injected though the same site to restore the vitreal volume post-sampling. This fluid can be sterile balanced salt solution or an appropriate drug.

RETINAL SURGERY

Retinal surgery is rarely undertaken by veterinary ophthalmologists, although various techniques using lasers are becoming more common. Retinal detachments are relatively common in dogs and on occasion can be successfully treated surgically. Possible indications for retinal or vitreoretinal surgery include detachments (e.g. following cataract surgery, vitreal degeneration, lens luxation or congenital abnormalities such as retinal dysplasia or collie eye anomaly) and the treatment of endophthalmitis. Techniques employed for retinal re-attachment surgery include the placement of scleral buckles, injection of heavy gases or oils into the posterior segment and total vitrectomy. The discussion of these techniques is beyond the scope of this book. However, we will discuss retinopexy surgery, which is the production of adhesions between the neurosensory retina and the underlying retinal pigment epithelium to prevent or limit retinal detachments. This is the most commonly undertaken retinal surgery in veterinary ophthalmology and has the advantages of being non-invasive and requiring less sophisticated instrumentation than the previously listed techniques.

Retinopexy can be performed using laser, usually a diode although several other types of laser can be successfully used (Table 5.2), or cryosurgery. The heat or cold cause adhesions, and 'spot weld' the retina in position. Both techniques can be used in a trans-scleral approach, usually prophylactically around the full circumference of the globe, 8–10 mm posterior to the limbus. The surgery is performed under general anaesthesia and is recommended prior to cataract surgery in cases at higher risk of retinal detachment post-cataract surgery—for example in cases with previous lens-induced uveitis, hypermature cataracts or in susceptible breeds such as the bichon frise. Ideally, a period of at least 2 weeks should be allowed between prophylactic trans-scleral retinopexy and elective cataract surgery. Retinopexy is also useful prior to lens luxation surgery since the risk of blinding retinal detachments is high following the removal of unstable lenses.

Laser retinopexy can also be used directly through the pupil by visualising the retina through an indirect ophthalmoscope attachment. This technique can be employed prophylactically but also around existing retinal detachments to prevent them spreading (e.g. with retinal dysplasia in the English springer spaniel). It is more successful in ventral retinal detachments since gravity does not continue to pull against the adhesions formed by the laser. With dorsal detachments, these gravitational forces are often greater than the strength of the adhesions such that the surgery fails and the detachment increases in size.

SUDDEN-ONSET BLINDNESS

The investigation and treatment of sudden-onset blindness can be a specialised area of ophthalmology. Clearly, some causes of sudden-onset blindness can be easily diagnosed and treated—for example, sudden-onset cataracts in diabetic dogs, retinal detachment in hypertensive cats or acute glaucoma. However, in some instances the animal rapidly loses vision with no obvious ophthalmic abnormalities being visible. Sudden acquired retinal degeneration (SARD) was discussed in Chapter 7. Although there is no treatment for this condition, it can be readily diagnosed by electroretinography, and the vast majority of dogs adjust very well. However, sometimes a patient will go suddenly blind, yet retain a normal electroretinogram. This indicates that the eye itself is functioning but there is a problem either with transmission of the visual information or with its central processing. Retrobulbar optic neuritis occurs when there is inflammation in the optic nerves which does not affect the optic discs such that ophthalmoscopically there is no evidence of this condition. Central lesions include neoplasia, inflammatory conditions, such as granulomatous meningoencephalitis (GME), and degenerative conditions (cognitive function disorders). Often, pupillary light reflexes can help to localise the lesion—they are normally abolished with optic nerve lesions, resulting in fixed dilated pupils, while some pupillary light reflex is usually retained in central disorders.

Once it has been confirmed that the eyes appear normal and electroretinography establishes that normal retinal function is present, more specialised investigation is warranted. A full neurological assessment is suggested together with advanced imaging techniques such as MRI or CT. The former is often more useful since it gives very good soft tissue definition. Cerebrospinal fluid samples might be taken if an infectious or multifocal inflammatory condition is suspected.

Treatment for retrobulbar optic neuritis usually involves systemic steroids and sometimes immunosuppressive agents such as azothioprine. Some dogs regain vision, while others do not and progress to develop optic atrophy. Similarly, chemotherapy or surgery for some types of brain neoplasia is possible, but the long-term prognosis for these patients must be guarded. Nurses are invaluable in providing guidance and support for both the patients and their owners.

ORBITAL SURGERY

Specialised orbital surgery includes the placement of orbital and intraocular prosthesis, and surgery of the retrobulbar space.

Orbital prostheses

An orbital prosthesis can be placed in the socket following routine enucleation and enhances the cosmetic appearance by preventing sinking of the skin into the hollow orbit after the eye is removed. They can be placed when cosmesis is of concern to the owner, but offer absolutely no benefit to the patient. They are most commonly used where intrascleral implants are contraindicated (e.g. following ocular neoplasia). Silicone is the most widely used material for the implant.

Intrascleral ocular prostheses

Intrascleral ocular prostheses are commonly used in the USA and Australia but rarely in Europe and the UK. The attitude of veterinary surgeons in the UK, as policed by the Royal College of Veterinary Surgeons, is that we must always consider the

welfare of the animal as our main priority—the wishes of the owner for a cosmetic appearance is much less important. However, as owners become even more cosmetically driven, the demand for these procedures is likely to increase. The technique is used for blind, painful eyes as an alternative to enucleation. It should not be used where neoplasia is suspected, nor in cats where there is a risk of intraocular sarcoma development.

The surgery is relatively straightforward. Under general anaesthesia, the eye is prepared routinely. A limbal- or fornix-based conjunctival flap is reflected to reveal the sclera, which is then incised approximately 5 mm behind the limbus for a length of 4–5 mm. A cyclodialysis spatula is used to bluntly dissect the uveal tissue from the sclera, and the entire contents of the globe are gently removed, including lens and retina. The tissue should be submitted for histological examination. Care must be taken not to damage the corneal endothelium. The hollow fibrous shell of cornea and sclera is carefully flushed to remove all fragments of tissue—haemorrhage usually subsides at this stage. The silicone implant can be injected using a special sphere-introducer. Different sizes are available—the other eye can be used as a measuring guide, or a sphere chosen 1–2 mm smaller than the surgical eye. Different colours are available to match the iris in the fellow eye if present. The sclera and overlying conjunctival flap are closed routinely. Postoperatively, there is often initial swelling and some discomfort. Systemic NSAIDs and topical antibiotic agents are required along with topical anti-inflammatory agents if indicated. Post-surgical nursing is routine.

Potential complications of intrascleral prostheses include infection, wound dehiscence and loss of the implant, regrowth of unidentified neoplasms and corneal ulceration. Owners must be aware that the 'eye' will not look normal—some corneal scarring is inevitable and the final ocular appearance cannot always be predicted. However, most owners are satisfied with the results of the procedure. It must be re-emphasised that the technique is performed purely for the benefit of the owner. The dog can still get corneal ulcers, eyelid problems and keratoconjunctivitis sicca, for example. One could argue that not only does the procedure confer no benefit to the patient but potentially can allow further suffering which would not occur if enucleation was performed.

Orbital surgery

Orbital surgery can be performed for retrobulbar space-occupying lesions, such as neoplasia and foreign bodies. Detailed imaging is suggested prior to any exploratory orbitotomy, and MRI or CT scans are preferable to ultrasonography and radiography. A lateral approach with removal of the zygomatic arch to gain access to the retrobulbar space is most commonly employed, and this approach can mean that the globe is not damaged and can be retained. In addition to a general soft-tissue surgical kit, orthopaedic equipment, such as rongeurs and drills, will be required by the surgeon. It is essential that the theatre nurse and surgeon discuss which instruments and equipment will be required since it will vary from case to case. Sometimes enucleation is required as well—for example, if a mass is closely adherent to the globe and optic nerve. The long-term outcome for orbital neoplasia is guarded since many tumours in this location are either locally invasive or metastatic.

EQUINE NURSING

Specialist knowledge is required when considering nursing the equine ophthalmology patient. The topic can be broadly divided into the following areas: safety, stabling, anatomical differences in horses, the common ocular problems encountered and ocular surgery. Equine anaesthesia is discussed in Chapter 6.

Safety

Obviously one must be aware of the potential for injury to personnel and damage to property by frightened horses, as well as the risks of them damaging themselves. Well-trained and experienced staff along with risk assessments are important safety measures.

Stabling

Horses might be hospitalised for intensive medical management—for example, to treat a severe uveitis or following surgery, such as repair of a corneal laceration. The importance of good hygiene cannot be overemphasised. Stables should be warm and dry with good drainage. They must be cleanable and able to be easily disinfected, with good ventilation, lighting and carefully planned food and water access. Fire risks must be assessed, including areas where straw and hay are kept, as well as wooden structures and so on. The environment must be as dust-free as possible. No sharp projections must be present within the stable (including window openings and food mangers which should be smooth). Hay racks should not be elevated—seeds and debris can easily fall into the eyes.

Anatomy of the equine eye

The most obvious differences from dogs and cats is the large size of the eyes and their lateral placement. The eye of the horse is the largest of all land mammals. Both the size and position make the equine eye more vulnerable to traumatic damage, and ocular trauma is one of the most common ophthalmic conditions encountered in the species. The lateral placement of the eyes offers a 300° field of view, ideal for the detection of predators. However, there are two small blind spots—one directly in front of the horse's nose and one directly behind its tail. This should be remembered when approaching horses, especially unfamiliar ones. Although equine ocular anatomy is basically very similar to dogs and cats (as described in Chapter 1), there are a few differences to point out. The eyeball itself is more oval than round in shape. The globe is well protected by a complete bony orbit. The pupil shape is of a horizontal oval, and along the dorsal aspect of the pupil there are several dark cystic structures attached to the pupillary edge—these are the granula iridica. They may assist in shading the ventral retina from excessive light levels. The retina is thinner than in dogs and cats, and the distribution of blood vessels is different, with arteries and veins only radiating for a few millimetres around the optic disc.

Ophthalmic examination of the horse

The ophthalmic examination of the horse follows same basic principles as discussed in Chapter 3. The animal is observed from a distance before a hands-on examination. Menace responses are not present in very young foals—they start to develop from 2 weeks of age. Assessment of the pupillary light reflexes requires two people since it is impossible to examine both eyes simultaneously. Thus, one person shines the light into one eye while the second observer notes any consensual constriction of the fellow pupil. If the stable or loose box cannot be darkened, the horse should be lead to a room which can be darkened sufficiently for an informative examination. If the horse is difficult to examine or in pain, it might be necessary to sedate the horse and consider an auriculopalpebral nerve block in order to complete the ophthalmic examination. This is particularly important if a traumatic injury has occurred—trying to force open the lids of a painfully lacerated eye could result in further ocular damage. This local nerve block abolishes the ability to blink, and the location for the injection of anaesthetic (such as lidocaine) is shown in Figure 6.12 (p. 101).

The eye is examined using the same equipment as detailed in Chapter 3. Mydriasis is recommended for a complete examination, although it often takes longer for tropicamide to take effect in horses. Two applications are usually necessary (10 minutes apart), and it takes 30 minutes before the pupils dilate. Tonometry using a Tonopen is possible. The Schiotz tonometer cannot be used since the cornea

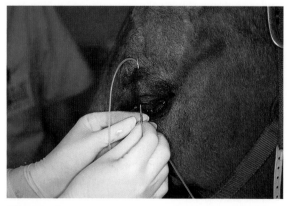

Fig. 8.15 Placement of a subpalpebral lavage system.

has to be horizontal for this instrument, and this is not feasible in awake horses! Gonioscopy is not necessary since the iridocorneal angle can be observed with simple illumination using a pen torch or Finhoff transilluminator in the horse. Nasolacrimal flushing can be easily performed in horses, but it is usually done in a retrograde manner—the nasal opening of the duct is cannulated and flushed up to the eye. The solution flushed from the ocular punctae must be carefully checked for fragments of foreign material, and samples taken for bacterial culture and sensitivity as required.

Medication

The application of drops is not easy in horses since their globes are so lateral with the cornea almost vertical—it is not easy to turn the head to one side to place the drop! Nor can one apply it from above as we advise in dogs and cats, except in Shetland ponies perhaps! As such, ointments are often chosen. However, drops are sometimes preferable (e.g. following corneal penetration). To apply them, a small amount (0.2 ml) should be drawn up into a 1 ml syringe. The needle is removed and the solution is sprayed into the eye. Topical anaesthesia is also best applied by this method.

If frequent or multiple topical medication is required, it might be easier to achieve through a lavage system. Horses often become head shy, particularly if the eye is painful, and this can make treatment difficult. The placement of a subpalpebral lavage system, or less frequently a nasolacrimal cannula, will make topical medication more straightforward. To place a subpalpebral lavage system, the horse is sedated and both auriculopalpebral (motor) and supraorbital (sensory) nerve blocks are placed. The supraorbital nerve block numbs the medial 2/3 of the upper eyelid (Fig. 6.13, p. 101). The commercially available silastic tubing of the lavage system is placed through the upper lid, along the dorsal fornix, and out of a second lid incision (Fig. 8.15). It is sutured via butterfly tapes into position, and if not pre-fenestrated, holes are put into the portion of tubing within the conjunctival fornix. The distal end of the tubing is taped behind the poll, or plaited into the mane, and an injection port attached to it

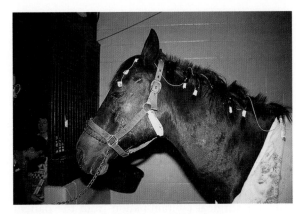

Fig. 8.16 Subpalpebral lavage system in situ.

(Fig. 8.16). Topical medication can then be injected through the tubing and is seen draining over the eye. Approximately 0.2–0.3 ml are used. Air or saline is used to flush the medication through the tubing. The substances should be injected gently so as not to startle the animal. The lavage system needs to be checked prior to each instillation to ensure that the ocular portion of the tubing remains tight within the upper fornix—if it loosens and slips down it can rub and cause corneal ulceration. When several different medications are being used topically, care must be taken to ensure that they are compatible and do not precipitate with each other, for example.

Horses can be light sensitive if eyes are painful or if atropine is used to treat them. As such, their stable must be shaded and bright lights avoided. Atropine can slow gut mobility and horses must be regularly checked since colic can occasionally develop in horses treated topically with atropine.

Self trauma can occur in horses, usually by rubbing against objects in the stable or on their forelegs. Cross-tying can prevent this or, alternatively, the use of head collars with protective eye cups can be considered (Fig. 6.14, p. 101).

Common equine ophthalmic problems

Trauma

Trauma is a very common cause of ocular damage in horses. All parts of the adnexa, globe and orbit can be involved. Injuries can range from a simple eyelid laceration, to more severe problems of corneal ulceration, corneal foreign body, full thickness perforation and iris prolapse, uveitis secondary to blunt trauma, and orbital fractures. General principles of first aid apply when dealing with injuries. The safety of all personnel as well as the horse must be considered. Details must be taken as to how the accident occurred and whether any other injuries have been incurred. Gentle pressure will ease bleeding from the lids, but this should not be excessive in case other ocular damage is present—for example, firm pressure on the closed lids could push a foreign body through the cornea. Sedation and nerve blocks should be considered to alleviate discomfort and prevent further damage. Once the nature of the injury has been fully assessed, the treatment plan can be drawn up.

Ulcers

Corneal ulcers in horses can range from simple ones which heal with a few days of topical antibiotics to deep stromal ulcers and descemetocoeles, as well as rapidly progressive melting ulcers. Intensive medical management or surgical debridement and conjunctival grafting under general anaesthesia might be required. Fungal infections are more common in horses than in small animals and can complicate ulcer healing. Corneal stromal abscesses are also seen in horses (Fig. 8.17).

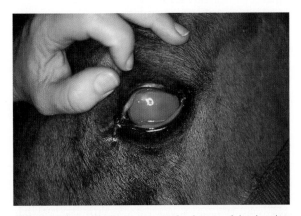

Fig. 8.17 Stromal abscess—note the increased lacrimation, corneal oedema, conjunctival hyperaemia and chemosis and yellow abscess just above the flash reflection.

Equine recurrent uveitis (ERU)

ERU is a common cause of blindness in horses. It is also known as periodic ophthalmia or moon blindness. Affected eyes are painful, with increased lacrimation, photophobia, blepharospasm, conjunctival hyperaemia and miosis. Aqueous flare or hypopyon and iridal swelling occur along with corneal oedema. Recurrent bouts lead to chronic scarring with synechiae, cataracts and secondary glaucoma. The disease is mainly immune-mediated but can be started by infectious agents such as leptospirosis. Medical therapy using topical steroids and atropine plus systemic NSAIDs is instigated. Relapses are frequent. The condition can be unilateral or bilateral. Occasionally extensive surgery with total vitrectomy is indicated in very severe cases.

Cataracts

Cataracts are seen less commonly in horses than in dogs. Inherited cataracts have been described in a few breeds, e.g. the Morgan horse. Congenital cataracts, sometimes with multiple ocular defects, can be seen occasionally in foals. However, ERU is the most common cause of equine cataracts. Surgery can be performed in some animals if vision is impaired.

Tumours

The most common equine ocular tumour is the squamous cell carcinoma, which can occur on the lids, including the third eyelid, the conjunctiva and the cornea. Cytology or biopsy will confirm the diagnosis. Excisional surgery together with cryosurgery, laser ablation or irradiation are common treatments. Intraocular tumours are sometimes seen, including melanoma and adenocarcinoma. Enucleation might be required.

Equine ocular surgery

Surgery in horses presents more of a challenge than in small animals simply as a result of their size. Simple procedures, such as suturing a small eyelid laceration or removing a superficial foreign body, can be performed in the standing horse.

Sedation is used together with an auriculopalpebral nerve block and appropriate sensory block, either with topical anaesthesia if the cornea needs to be desensitised, or via a supraorbital nerve block if lid sensation needs to be abolished. Surgical preparation of the operation site is performed in the same way as in small animals. Radiography can be performed in awake or sedated horses (e.g. to investigate orbital fractures).

More complex procedures require general anaesthesia (Table 8.12). Details on equine anaesthesia are included in Chapter 6. There are increased risks for surgical contamination from the patient itself compared to small animals—meticulous preoperative preparation is necessary to minimise this. Induction and recovery boxes must have padded walls and non-slip floors, along with overhead hoists to move the anaesthetised patient into theatre where a mobile hydraulic theatre table is present. The patient will normally be placed in lateral recumbency. The down-side eye must be carefully protected—it is very exposed and easily damaged. In addition to padding around the head, lubricants should be applied to the eye. Instrument kits for ophthalmic surgery in horses will be similar to those for small animals. Many

Table 8.12 Surgical procedures necessitating general anaesthesia in the horse

Condition	Procedure
Corneal laceration	Suture to repair
Corneal foreign body	Surgical removal
Deep or melting ulcer	Conjunctival graft
Cataract	Remove by phacoemulsification
Equine recurrent uveitis	Vitrectomy ± cataract removal sometimes used along with medical management
Orbital fracture	Stabilise if necessary (wire or plate), remove sequestered bone fragments
Severe ocular trauma	Enucleate
Intraocular neoplasia	Enucleate

procedures can be performed using magnifying head loupes, but an operating microscope is necessary for intraocular surgery such as cataract removal.

Nursing horses with ocular problems will include general hospital monitoring together with topical and systemic medication as detailed above. Owners must be competent at medicating their horse. Often two people are required, one to hold the horse while the other administers the topical treatment. If the owner is not able to arrange for this, possibly several times daily, then the horse might be better off staying in the hospital until off topical treatment.

BIBLIOGRAPHY AND FURTHER READING

Barnett KC, et al. Equine Ophthalmology. 2nd edn. Edinburgh: WB Saunders; 2004.

Coumbe KM, ed. Equine veterinary nursing manual. Oxford: Blackwell Science; 2001.

Gelatt KN, Gelatt JP. Handbook of small animal ophthalmic surgery. Volumes 1 and 2. Oxford: Pergamon; 1994.

Gelatt KN. Veterinary ophthalmology. 3rd edn. Philadelphia: Lippincott Williams & Wilkins; 1999.

Lane DR, Cooper B, eds. Veterinary nursing. 3rd edn. Oxford: Butterworth Heinemann; 2003.

Moore AH, ed. BSAVA manual of advanced veterinary nursing. Gloucester: British Small Animal Veterinary Association; 1999.

Petersen-Jones S, Crispin S, eds. BSAVA manual of small animal ophthalmology. 2nd edn. Gloucester: British Small Animal Veterinary Association; 2002.

Special issue: ocular surgery. Veterinary Ophthalmology 2004; Vol. 7, No. 5.

9 Inherited eye disease in dogs

INTRODUCTION

Unfortunately, inherited eye diseases are very common in dogs. They are less of a problem in cats, but with the increase in popularity of unusual pedigree cats the incidence of inherited ocular conditions can be expected to increase. Inherited problems can be congenital or develop later in life, and can have various effects on the animal, ranging from no pain or effect on vision to severe pain and blindness. To try to reduce the incidence of these conditions, testing schemes have been set up in various countries. The UK scheme is discussed in detail below, with brief mention of other control programmes elsewhere in the world. The World Small Animal Veterinary Association (WSAVA) has an Hereditary Defects Committee, and discussions on standardisation among testing in different countries with the aim of producing an internationally recognised scheme are in progress (Table 9.1).

THE BVA/KC/ISDS SCHEME

A scheme is run by the British Veterinary Association (BVA), Kennel Club (KC) and International Sheep Dog Society (ISDS). The scheme was set up over 30 years ago, initially as a screening programme for progressive retinal atrophy (PRA). Now 11 recognised inherited diseases in almost 50 breeds are certified. In addition, further conditions and breeds are 'under investigation', i.e. clinical evidence suggests an inherited basis but more research needs undertaking to confirm whether the disease is inherited in that particular breed. The purpose of the eye testing scheme is to provide a service to breeders and dog owners to help reduce the incidence of inherited disorders.

The BVA runs the scheme and processes the results which are passed on to the Kennel Club for publication. Breeds and conditions are under constant review by the Eye Panel Working Party. The lists of breeds certified under the scheme are updated twice a year in January and July. The Scheme is voluntary—about 13 000 dogs are tested annually. Its success can be demonstrated in the Border collie, where strict controls by ISDS have resulted in a decrease in the incidence of PRA from 14% to less than 0.25%.

Panellists have either a Royal College of Veterinary Surgeons (RCVS) certificate or diploma

Table 9.1 Contact details for eye testing schemes

British Veterinary Association 7 Mansfield Street London W1G 9NQ England Tel 44 (0)207 636 6541 www. bva.co.uk	Runs the UK BVA/KC/ISDS scheme Will provide a list of panellists plus information sheets for breeders and details of breeds and conditions currently certified
The Kennel Club 1–5 Clarges Street Piccadilly London W1J 8AB Tel 44 (0) 870 606 6750 www.the-kennel-club.org.uk	Publishes the results of eye tests (both affected and non-affected) in quarterly breed records supplement
European College of Veterinary Ophthalmologists www.ecvo.org	Oversees members of panel Provides details of the examination Provides lists of panellists in participating countries
Canine Eye Registration Foundation Purdue University West Lafayette IN 47907 USA www.vmdb.org/cerf.html	Runs CERF scheme Provides information for breeders Registers dogs free from eye disease
Optigen llc Cornell Business and Technology Park 767 Warren Road Suite 300 Ithaca, New York Tel 607 257 0301 Fax 607 257 0353 www.optigen.com	Provides DNA testing for a wide range of inherited ocular disease

in veterinary ophthalmology, and an assessment on the theory and practice of the scheme is necessary before new panellists are appointed. Full examination of all dogs includes slit lamp biomicroscopy, and indirect and direct ophthalmoscopy after mydriasis. Gonioscopy is performed as an additional test in breeds affected with goniodysgenesis (and is performed before the routine eye test if both are being undertaken).

Adult dogs are tested and issued with a certificate of eye examination. The certificate issued is in several parts: the top section refers to the dog, the middle section has any abnormalities described in words and diagrams, and the bottom section classes the dog as affected or unaffected for the conditions recognised in that breed. Owners and breeders must supply the original Kennel Club registration certificate for the dog to enable the eye test to be performed and the certificate issued. The panellist stamps and signs the KC registration document

when the certificate is issued. The top white copy is kept by the owner, the blue copy goes to the BVA, the panellist keeps the yellow copy, while the dog's usual veterinary surgeon gets the bottom pink copy. An appeals procedure is in place for owners to seek a second opinion from another panellist if they are unhappy with the result.

Litter screening is performed for congenital diseases. Breeders are encouraged to present whole litters for testing. Puppies must be less than 12 weeks old for litter screening. The results of litter tests are not published by the Kennel Club but are used by the breeders to select animals for future breeding.

OTHER EYE TESTING SCHEMES

The European scheme

The Eye Scheme of the European College of Veterinary Ophthalmologists (ECVO) has been recently set up. Countries using the scheme include the Netherlands, Norway, Denmark, Finland, Germany and Switzerland. The UK retains its separate scheme (although the UK Kennel Club does recognise the certificates issued under the ECVO scheme). The long-established scheme run by the Swedish Kennel Club also remains separate. It is likely that in time more countries will adopt the European scheme. Panellists issuing certificates must be ECVO diplomats or be members of the relevant national eye testing scheme who have undergone stringent examination by the ECVO. At present there is no pan-European collation of the results—the breed or kennel clubs for the individual countries collect the results and offer advice regarding breeding.

The Hereditary Eye Scheme in the USA

Certification for inherited eye disease in the USA is run by the Canine Eye Registration Foundation (CERF). The organisation was founded by a group of pedigree dog breeders who were concerned about inherited eye disease, and the aims of organisation are to 'accomplish the goal of elimination of heritable eye disease in all pure-bred dogs by forming a centralised, national registry'. CERF examinations are performed by ophthalmologists who are board-certified (i.e. Diplomats) of the American College of Veterinary Ophthalmologists (ACVO). CERF gathers all the data from the certificates, and animals which are free from eye disease can be registered with CERF (and breeders can advertise as such). CERF works closely with the genetics committee of the ACVO, and recommendations regarding breeding are provided by the committee.

Eye testing in Australia

As yet there is no official eye testing scheme in Australia. However, specialists in ophthalmology (i.e. those veterinary surgeons who have attained Fellowship of the Australian College of Veterinary Science [FACVS] in ophthalmology, or are Diplomats from the USA, UK or Europe) examine and issue certificates for breeders, as well as offering advice regarding the significance of any findings.

BVA/KC/ISDS SCHEME

In this section, the different inherited eye diseases are considered—mostly those certified under the UK scheme but with mention of other conditions, such as entropion, which are associated with general facial conformation. It is suggested that responsible breeding programmes should recognise these exaggerated facial features and selectively breed away from them. For example, in the CERF scheme it is advised that in English bulldogs with entropion, breeding is not recommended. The conditions below are only described briefly since they are mentioned in more detail in the chapters on general ophthalmological conditions and specialist procedures. Some repetition is inevitable but is included for ease of reference.

Congenital inherited diseases

Multiple ocular defects (MOD)

A combination of microphthalmos, cataract, retinal dysplasia, nystagmus and persistent pupillary membrane is seen from time to time in dogs. The condition is bilateral but not always symmetrical. Breeds under investigation include bloodhound, cavalier King Charles spaniel, rough collie, Doberman, old English sheepdog, golden retriever and English cocker spaniel.

Persistent pupillary membrane (PPM)

Small and insignificant remnants of the pupillary membrane are commonly seen in dogs. More severe remnants can occasionally affect vision. Strands of tissue arise from the iris and can remain as tags from the iris or can adhere to the anterior lens capsule or the back of the cornea. Focal opacities are present at the site of adherence. Affected breeds include the basenji, bullmastiff, English cocker spaniel and Siberian husky.

Congenital cataract (CC)

Congenital cataracts are most often positioned in the centre of the lens and rarely progress. Thus, as the animal grows vision can actually improve as normal lens material is deposited around the central opacity. Congenital cataracts can occur in isolation or in conjunction with other defects—part of the MOD syndrome. Affected breeds are the miniature schnauzer, old English sheepdog, golden retriever and West Highland white terrier.

Persistent hyperplastic primary vitreous (PHPV)

This is seen in the Doberman and Staffordshire bull terrier. An abnormality occurs in the differentiation of the posterior lens capsule, and persistent hyaloid vessels can be present. Although bilateral, there can be a significant difference between the two eyes. The affect on vision is extremely variable.

Collie eye anomaly (CEA)

This is seen in rough and smooth collies, Shetland sheep dogs, Border collies, and has recently been described in the Lancashire heeler. It has also been documented in the Australian shepherd dog, although not in the UK. Diagnosis is best performed at 6 weeks of age. The pathognomic sign is choroidal hypoplasia lateral to the optic disc. The choroidal vessels in the area are abnormal in form and distribution with fewer, larger vessels and reduced pigment in the retinal pigment epithelium, allowing exposure of the sclera (and a pale patch). This can be difficult to detect in merle-coloured animals which have non-pigmented fundi normally. About $\frac{1}{3}$ of cases also have colobomas (holes or absence of tissue), usually on the optic or very close to it. Retinal detachment and intraocular haemorrhage are less common but result in blindness in the affected eye.

Dogs affected with choroidal hypoplasia only can sometimes appear ophthalmoscopically to 'go normal'. Here the retinal pigment epithelium covers the underlying pathology as the animal matures, although phenotypically the animal is still affected.

CEA is thought to have an autosomal recessive inheritance.

Retinal dysplasia (RD)

Retinal dysplasia is a congenital disease in which the retina fails to differentiate normally. There are two main types—multifocal (MRD) or total (TRD). The former is generally less severe and manifests as multiple folds within the retina which can be detected at 6 weeks of age. Affected breeds include the cavalier King Charles spaniel, rottweiler, American cocker and English springer spaniels, and golden and Labrador retrievers (see Table 7.16, p. 130). Geographic retinal dysplasia is the term used to describe severe forms of the multifocal disease. In most animals the affect on vision is minimal but in some cases the retina can detach rendering the dog blind (e.g. in English springer spaniels).

A more severe form of retinal dysplasia is seen in Sealyham and Bedlington terriers plus Labrador retrievers. This total retinal dysplasia leaves affected dogs blind due to retinal non-attachment.

Goniodysgenesis (G)

Abnormalities in the differentiation of the pectinate ligaments and drainage angles can predispose to primary glaucoma. Screening from 6 months of age can eliminate affected dogs from the breeding pool. Breeds affected include the basset hound, flat coated retriever, Siberian husky, most types of spaniel, great Dane and Dandie Dinmont terrier (Table 7.12, p. 126). Many other breeds are 'under investigation' or are assumed to suffer from inherited goniodysgenesis in other countries.

Primary glaucoma is a bilateral condition and is very difficult to treat successfully. Acute glaucoma must be treated as an emergency and the second eye is always at risk.

Non-congenital inherited ocular disease

Eyelid

Adnexal abnormalities have a breed-related presentation and thus must have an inherited component. However, they do not form part of the BVA/KC/ISDS scheme. Entropion is the term given to the rolling in of the lid margin towards the cornea. Both eyes are usually affected and it causes chronic irritation with increased lacrimation and blepharospasm. Chronic entropion leads to inflammation of the cornea (keratitis) and ulceration.

Several breeds suffer from entropion, including the Shar-pei, chow chow, Labrador retriever and spaniels of various types. Advice to owners of affected breeds is limited to suggesting that affected individuals are not used for breeding. However, this is difficult in some breeds where virtually every individual appears affected to some degree!

Ectropion is rolling out of the lid. It is most common in breeds with loose skin such as basset hounds, English cocker spaniels and bloodhounds. It does not usually cause discomfort but can allow accumulation of debris in the lower conjunctival fold (fornix), predisposing to chronic conjunctivitis and recurrent infections. Giant breeds in particular can suffer from a combination of entropion and ectropion—the so called diamond eye typified by the Saint Bernard, great Dane and clumber spaniel. Surgical correction of these lid abnormalities can be challenging.

Problems with the third eyelid include scrolling of the cartilage and prolapse of the nictitans gland. Both require surgical correction and are potentially bilateral. Affected individuals should not be used for breeding.

Eyelashes

Eyelash (cilia) disorders are also quite common and are breed-related—this means that they are more common in certain breeds of dogs but the actual inheritance has not been worked out. Like eyelid conditions, they are not considered as part of the UK testing scheme. The most common form of lash disorder is distichiasis—eyelashes growing from the opening of the meibomian glands on the lid margin itself. It is very common in cocker spaniels, miniature long haired dachshunds and poodles (miniature and toy). A more severe form of eyelash abnormality is the ectopic cilium. This is an eyelash which grows through the lid to emerge on the inner lid conjunctiva directing straight at the cornea. Each time the dog blinks this little sharp hair rubs up and down on

the cornea. It is easy to see how persistent or recurrent ulceration are common. Good light and magnification are necessary to visualise the cilia. Flat coated retrievers are most commonly affected.

Cornea

Corneal lipidosis is a bilateral inherited condition in which opacities appear in the central cornea. They are found in the anterior stroma and are not associated with discomfort or visual disturbance and appear in early adulthood. Affected breeds include cavalier King Charles spaniels, Siberian huskies, Shetland sheepdogs and rough collies, and more recently golden retrievers. However, there are many other causes for corneal lipid deposits (hypothyroidism, hyperlipidaemia, Cushing's disease, etc.), so a thorough general clinical examination is mandatory to rule out systemic disease.

Lens

There are two main conditions affecting the lens which can be inherited, namely cataract (HC) and primary lens luxation (PLL).

A cataract is an opacity of the lens. There are many causes of cataract, e.g. post-inflammatory or traumatic, metabolic (mainly from diabetes mellitus), senile and of course hereditary. When deciding whether a cataract is hereditary we must consider the location of the cataract within the lens, the breed and the age of dog. Many breeds are affected with cataracts which tend to affect specific parts of the lens and progress in a set pattern. Hereditary cataract can be congenital as mentioned previously or occur later in life (e.g. golden retriever or Boston terrier). Age of onset and rate of progression vary according to the breed—for example, many retriever cataracts do not progress to affect vision but almost all progress to blindness in the Staffordshire bull terrier. Table 7.9 (p. 123) details inherited cataracts in dogs in the UK.

Primary lens luxation (PLL) occurs when the lens slips out of its normal position due to zonular rupture. It is common in terriers—the Jack Russell, Sealyham and fox terriers together with the border collie and Shar-pei (Table 7.10, p. 124).

The condition is bilateral, although one eye usually is affected before the other. It manifests in young adulthood. Subluxated lenses can be detected by signs of iris wobble, strands of vitreous in the anterior chamber and shallowing or deepening of the anterior chamber itself (depending which way the lens is moving).

Retina

The progressive retinal atrophies (PRA) are a collection of diseases which affect many breeds. They can be divided into generalised PRA (GPRA), which results in total blindness, and central PRA (CPRA)—now correctly called retinal pigment epitheial dystrophy (RPED)—which does not always lead to total vision loss. GPRA can be due to photoreceptor dysplasia, where the retina never forms properly, or due to photoreceptor degeneration. The different forms affect dogs at different ages with different rates of progression, but all types result in degeneration of the retina and secondary cataract formation. Typically, there is a progression from poor night vision to loss of day vision over months to years in early middle age (as seen in the toy and miniature poodle, English cocker spaniel and Labrador retriever). Table 7.17 (p. 131) lists the breeds currently certified under the UK scheme, together with the age when the ophthalmoscopic signs can be seen. Ophthalmo-scopically, tapetal hyper-reflectivity and blood vessel attenuation are noted, followed by patchy depigmentation of the non-tapetal fundus. Optic atrophy and total retinal degeneration result. The lesions are bilateral and symmetrical. Owners often notice the secondary cataracts and attribute the loss of vision to these. There is no treatment. Hence, control through regular eye tests is essential until more DNA blood tests are available which detect affected, carrier and clear dogs.

Retinal pigment epithelial dystrophy (RPED) is an ocular manifestation of a metabolic defect, and affected animals usually have low serum vitamin E. Ophthalmoscopic signs include light-brown lipopigment foci in the tapetal fundus, which enlarge and coalesce with irregular hyper-reflective patches in between. Vascular attenuation and optic atrophy are variable. Dietary supplementation with vitamin E can arrest progression. The cocker spaniel appears most frequently affected and Table 7.19 (p. 132) lists the breeds currently certified.

Optic nerve hypoplasia (ONH)

Failure of the normal development of the optic nerve results in hypoplasia. Affected animals have reduced vision or are blind. Miniature and toy poodles and miniature long-haired dachshunds are affected.

Appendix 1
Ocular emergencies

In this section we aim to briefly outline some ophthalmic emergencies and discuss the immediate management required. Further details of each condition can be found in the chapters on general and specialist ophthalmic procedures.

Proptosis

Proptosis or prolapse of the eyeball is a genuine emergency. It is most common in brachycephalic patients. Trauma is usually the inciting cause (e.g. a fight with another dog). The immediate first aid requirements are to keep the eyeball moist and to prevent further damage to it. Thus, when an owner telephones for advice they should be told to keep the eye wet (a damp cloth is ideal) until they arrive at the surgery. Initial assessment should check the degree of damage—for example, if the optic nerve has been severed or the globe ruptured then enucleation is advised. If the globe can be salvaged, and the patient is suitable for general anaesthesia, the eye can be repositioned as outlined in Chapter 7.

Blunt trauma

Blunt trauma to the eye can occur due to a variety of causes (e.g. a road traffic accident, being kicked or hit by a ball). The patient should be carefully examined for injuries to other parts of the body. It might be necessary to sedate the patient to enable a thorough ocular examination. The eye can be gently irrigated with sterile saline to remove debris before assessing if the globe has ruptured. Hyphaema will alert the observer to this possibility. A corneal rupture should be relatively easy to detect, but if a posterior scleral rupture has occurred it might be necessary to perform ocular ultrasonography. If the globe has ruptured it should be assessed to see if surgical repair is feasible—if not then early enucleation is advised. Radiography might also be needed to check for skull fractures. Subconjunctival haemorrhages can be marked following trauma and, providing the globe itself is not badly damaged, they tend to resorb in 7–10 days.

Corneal injuries

Emergencies which involve the cornea include lacerations, foreign bodies (especially if perforated), deep corneal ulcers (such as a descemetocoele), melting ulcers and chemical burns. In general the patient will present with a painful eye, usually with a moderate ocular discharge. This will be serous or blood-stained if a full thickness laceration has occurred but is more likely to be mucopurulent in the case of a deep or melting ulcer. Emergency referral should be considered if there is any doubt about management.

Acute uveitis

Acute uveitis can be unilateral or bilateral. The patient might be systemically unwell. The patient will present with a sudden-onset painful eye, with corneal oedema and marked episcleral congestion. There might be a reduction in vision, or even total blindness. Further details are in Chapter 7.

Acute glaucoma

Sudden-onset glaucoma is both a sight-threatening and potentially eye-threatening condition, and its early recognition is essential if successful management is to ensue. The presentation is similar to acute uveitis—a red, cloudy, painful eye with reduced vision. Tonometry is mandatory. If there is any doubt about the diagnosis, urgent referral should be considered. Further details are present in Chapters 7 and 8.

Acute lens luxation

As with both acute uveitis and glaucoma, a patient with an acute lens luxation, assuming that the lens has dislocated into the anterior chamber, will present with a red, cloudy, painful eye and reduced vision in the affected eye. The condition can be readily diagnosed with a careful ophthalmic examination and referral for surgery should be considered as an emergency.

Sudden-onset blindness

There are several causes for sudden-onset blindness, including retinal detachments, sudden acquired retinal degeneration, and hypertensive retinopathy, as well as causes unrelated to the eye itself, such as a brain tumour. A careful clinical and ophthalmic examination is essential to reach the diagnosis. Referral should be considered for further investigation if necessary.

Acute exophthalmos

Acute exophthalmos, or protrusion of the eye, should be treated as an emergency to prevent damage to the eye, such as corneal ulceration due to exposure, or permanent damage to the optic nerve as a result of stretching and pressure from the swelling. Animals are usually in significant discomfort and might be systemically unwell (e.g. pyrexic and lethargic). Retrobulbar abscesses and cellulitis are the most commonly encountered causes, and once diagnosed can usually be managed fairly easily.

Emergency ophthalmic nursing

The role of the nurse in an ophthalmic emergency often begins with telephone advice to the client. This might include cold compresses for acute exophthalmos, or keeping the patient very quiet until examined for a potential foreign body. The duty veterinary surgeon should alert the nurse to the suspected problem as soon as possible such that any appropriate equipment and instruments can be prepared if required. The patient will need gentle restraint for examination, possibly with sedation, and the nurse can assist with this. Once the diagnosis has been reached, a management plan can be drawn up. This might involve referral, in which case the nurse can contact the referral specialist and fax all relevant history in advance. If the patient is to be managed at the surgery, the nurse can liaise with other members of the team such that all medical and surgical procedures are undertaken as soon as possible to provide the best prognosis for the patient. Owners should be given a realistic expected outcome following the emergency and should be calmly reassured that all is being done for their pet. The nurse has an important role in communicating with owners, especially in emergency situations when they are likely to be upset and might not fully understand the problem and its implications. It is good protocol for the nurse to telephone the owners as soon as the patient has stabilised, or as soon as the surgery is completed, to set their minds at rest and let them know that the ophthalmologist will contact them shortly with further details.

Appendix 2
Causes of blindness in dogs and cats

The most common causes of blindness will be listed here, divided into those which are sudden in onset and those which occur more gradually. For futher details on each condition refer to Chapters 7 and 8. In addition, for each condition I have highlighted whether dogs or cats are usually affected.

	Dogs	Cats
Sudden blindness		
Glaucoma	●	
Retinal detachment	●	●
Hypertensive retinopathy	○	●
Severe uveitis	●	●
Sudden acquired retinal degeneration	●	
Hyphaema/other intraocular haemorrhage	●	●
Sudden-onset cataract due to diabetes mellitus	●	
Severe trauma	●	●
Proptosis	●	○
Optic neuritis	●	
Central mass	●	○
Central anoxia/hypoxia	●	●
Gradual onset		
Severe keratitis (such as chronic superficial keratitis)	●	
Pigmentary keratitis	●	
Corneal oedema	●	○
Cataract	●	●
Chronic uveitis	●	●
Chronic glaucoma	●	○
Chorioretinitis	●	○
Progressive retinal atrophy (PRA)	●	○

● – Common ○ – Less frequent Blank – rarely encountered

Appendix 3
Suppliers of ophthalmic surgical products

The companies listed below are a small selection of the many suppliers of ophthalmic instruments, equipment and disposable items. The list is not exhaustive but should provide a good reference point for sourcing supplies. Many of the companies listed also have overseas offices and will ship worldwide. For more companies, including manufacturers of phacoemulsification machines for example, the human ophthalmic journals include many advertisers.

Company	Products
UK Companies	
Altomed Ltd 2 Witney Way Boldon Business Park Tyne & Wear NE35 0PE Tel 0191–519–0111 Fax 0191–519–0283 www.altomed.com	Ophthalmic surgical instruments
Animalcare Ltd Common Road Dunnington York YO19 5RU Tel 01904–487–687 Fax 01904–487–611 www.animalcare.co.uk	Keeler ophthalmoscopes Slit lamps Surgical instruments
BD Ophthalmic Products 21 Between Towns Road Cowley Oxford OX4 3LY Tel 01865–748–844 Fax 01865–781–627 www.bd.com/ophthalmology	Surgical drapes Intraocular cannulae Cataract instruments Knives

Company	Products
Collton Hailsham Ltd 57 The drive Hailsham East Sussex BN27 3HW Tel 01373–440–433 Fax 01323–440–433 www.colltonhailsham.co.uk	Ophthalmic surgical instruments
Dixey Instruments 5 High Street Brixworth Northants NN6 9DD Tel 01604–882–480 Fax 01604–882–488 www.dixeyinstruments.com	Ophthalmic surgical instruments
Duckworth & Kent Ltd Terence House 7 Marquis Business Centre Royston Road Baldock Herts SG7 6XL Tel 01462–893–254 Fax 01462–896–288 www.duckworth-and-kent.com	Ophthalmic surgical instruments
Hales Veterinary Speciality Products PO Box 1, Rosemary Lane Whitchurch Shrops SY14 7WF Tel 01948–780–624 Fax 01948–780–623 www.sjhjales.co.uk	Diagnostic equipment Contact lenses Instruments
Spectrum Ophthalmics Fernbank House Springwood Way Macclesfield SK10 2XA Tel 01625 618–816 Fax 01625–619–959 www.spectrum-uk.co.uk	Wide range of disposables for ocular surgery
Vision matrix 31 East Parade Harrogate HG1 5LQ Tel 01423–705–058 Fax 01423–705–056 www.visionmatrix.co.uk	Variety of equipment including: Instrument trays Cataract disposables Intraocular lenses
John Weiss & Son Ltd 89-90 Alston Drive Bradwell Abbey Milton Keynes MK13 9HF Tel 01908–318–017 Fax 01908–318–708 www.johnweiss.com	Ophthalmic surgical instruments

Company	Products
Carl Zeiss Ltd 15–20 Woodfield Road Welwyn Garden City Herts AL7 1JQ Tel 01707–871–200 Fax 01707–330–237 www.zeiss.co.uk	Operating microscopes

European Companies

Acri.tec Neuendorfstraffe 20a 16761 Heningsdorf Tel 49 3302–2026920 Fax 49 3302–2026915 www.acritec.de	Disposables for ocular surgery Intraocular lenses Instruments
Dioptrix 13 Rue D'Ariane 31240 L'Union, France Tel 33–534–301244 Fax 33–561–610995 www.dioptrix.com	Intraocular lenses Cataract disposables Ultrasound machines
Eickemeyer Eltastrasse 8 78532 Tuttlingen Germany Tel 49–7461–96580–0 Fax 49–7461–96580–90 www.eickemeyer.de	Welch Allyn ophthalmoscopes Radiosurgery equipment Range of diagnostic and surgical instruments

US companies

Dan Scott & Associates 235 Luke Court Westerville OH 43081 Tel 614–890–0370 Fax 614–818–9330 www.danscotrandassociates.com	Tonopen tonometer Blood pressure monitors Keeler and Welch Allyn distributors
Eye Care Distributors International 10769 Oak Lake Way Suite 100 Boca Raton Fl 33498 Tel 561–883–3769 Fax 561–488–2279	Surgical products Cataract products
I-Med Pharma 1601 St Regis Blvd Montreal Quebec H9B 3H7 Canada Tel 514–685–8118 Fax 514–685–8998 www.imedpharma.com	Surgical instruments Surgical disposables

Company	Products
Iridex 1212 Terra Bella Avenue Mountain View Ca 94043 Tel 650–940–4700 Fax 650–940–4710 www.iridex.com	Diode lasers and accessories
J C Enterprises 22971 Triton Way Suite E Laguna Hills CA 92653 Tel 949–643–5067 Fax 949–831–6534 www.ophthalmicqdp.com	Full range of ophthalmic instruments and equipment including cataract equipment
Ocularvision Inc 575 Farmland Drive Buelton California 93427 Tel 805–688–4400 Fax 805–688–5126 www.ocularvision.com	Intraocular lenses
Sontec Instruments Inc 7248 South Tucson Way Englewood CO 80112 Tel 303–790–9411 Fax 303–792–2606 www.sontecinstruments.com	Surgical and ophthalmic instruments
Australian companies	
Designs for Vision 1 Denison Street Camperdown NSW 2050 Tel 02–9550–6966 Fax 02–9550–3853 www.dfv.com.au	General ophthalmic equipment Operating microscopes Intraocular lenses
Device Technologies Australia Unit 8, 25 Frenchs Forest Road Frenchs Forest NSW 2086 Tel 02–9975–5755 Fax 02–9975–5711 www.objectvision.com	Wide range of ophthalmic equipment Distributors for many companies including Heine, Haag–Streit
Spectrum Ophthalmics PO Box 2188 Fountain Gate VIC 3805 Tel 03–9705–0553 Fax 03–8790–5114	Wide range of disposables for ocular surgery

Glossary

Accommodation
ability to focus by changing the shape of the lens.

Acuity
visual ability to differentiate shapes—visual sharpness.

Adnexa
eyelids, conjunctiva, lacrimal glands and orbital contents.

Anisocoria
difference in size of the two pupils.

Anterior chamber
the fluid-filled space between the cornea and iris/lens.

Aphakia
absence of lens.

Aqueous flare
clouding to anterior chamber due to increased protein in the aqueous humour.

Aqueous humour
clear fluid filling the anterior chamber.

Area centralis
area of the retina with highest cone density, found dorsolateral to the optic disc.

Asteroid hyalosis
solid bodies of calcium–lipid complex found in normal vitreous gel.

Astigmatism
refractive error caused by asymmetry of the corneal curvature.

Blepharitis
inflammation of the eyelids.

Blepharospasm
spasm of the orbicularis oculi muscle causing increased blink rate.

Blood–ocular barrier
functional barrier between the general circulation and the eye.

Blood–aqueous barrier
functional barrier between the general circulation and the anterior chamber.

Blood–retinal barrier
functional barrier between the general circulation and the retina.

Canthotomy
incision of the canthus.

Capsulorhexis
removal of a piece of the anterior lens capsule by controlled tearing.

Caruncle
piece of skin at the medial canthus (can be haired).

Cataract
opacity of the lens and/or lens capsule.

Chalazion
chronic inflammatory granuloma of meibomian gland.

Chemosis
swelling (oedema) of the conjunctiva.

Choroid
the posterior uveal tract between the retina and sclera.

Choroidal hypoplasia
congenital lack of normal development of the choroid seen in collie eye anomaly.

Ciliary body
part of the uveal tract between the iris and choroid.

Collie eye anomaly (CEA)
congenital, inherited condition with choroidal hypoplasia as pathognomic ophthalmoscopic sign.

Coloboma
a congenital hole or absence of tissue.

Cone
photoreceptor specialised for daylight vision.

Congenital
present at birth.

Conjunctiva
mucous membrane lining the eyelids and front of the eye (apart from over the cornea).

Conjunctivitis
inflammation of the conjunctiva.

Cornea
transparent portion of the outer layer of the eyeball.

Cyclodialysis
glaucoma surgery involving the creation of a fistula between the anterior chamber and sclera.

Cyclophotocoagulation
laser surgery to destroy the ciliary body.

Cyclocryotherapy
freezing surgery to destroy the ciliary body.

Cycloplegia
paralysis of the ciliary body muscle (usually drug-induced).

Dacryocystitis
inflammation of the lacrimal gland (and usually nasolacrimal duct).

Dermoid
congenital skin growth in abnormal location.

Descemet's membrane
thin elastic layer of the cornea between the stroma and endothelium.

Descemetocoele
deep ulcer with protrusion of Descemet's membrane.

Distichiasis
aberrant cilia along the lid margin.

Dysplasia
abnormal development.

Ectopic cilia
abnormal cilia growing through palpebral conjunctiva.

Ectropion
out-turning of the eyelid.

Electroretinogram (ERG)
the recording of electrical responses in the retina when stimulated by light.

Endophthalmitis
inflammation of the internal structures of the eye.

Enophthalmos
a sunken eye.

Entropion
in-rolling of the eyelid margin.

Enucleation
surgical removal of the eyeball.

Epiphora
tear overflow

Exophthalmos
abnormal protrusion of the eye.

Fornix
junction between the palpebral and bulbar conjunctiva.

Fundus
the posterior layers of the eye as viewed by an ophthalmoscope.

Glaucoma
raised intraocular pressure causing damage to optic nerve.

Globe
eyeball.

Goniodysgenesis
congenital malformation of the iridocorneal angle.

Goniolens
plastic lens used for gonioscopy.

Gonioscopy
technique to examine the iridocorneal angle.

Granula iridica
darkly pigmented iris extensions at the dorsal pupil of the equine eye.

Heterochromia iridis
more than one colour to the iris or having a different colour in each eye.

Hordeolum
stye.

Hyalitis
inflammation of the vitreous.

Hyaloid vessels
blood vessels present between the optic disc and lens during embryogenesis.

Hypermetropia
long-sightedness.

Hyphaema
haemorrhage in the anterior chamber.

Hypopyon
white blood cells (pus) in the anterior chamber.

Hypotony
low intraocular pressure.

Intracameral
into the anterior chamber.

Iridencleisis
glaucoma surgery using a hole in the iris to act as wick drawing aqueous into the subconjunctival space.

Iridocorneal angle
angle between the iris and the cornea where aqueous drainage occurs.

Iris
coloured portion of the uveal tract in front of the lens with the pupil in its centre.

Iris bombé
adhesions between the iris and anterior lens capsule extending around the full pupil circumference.

Keratitis
inflammation of the cornea.

Keratoconjunctivitis sicca
dry eye—lack of aqueous tear production.

Keratectomy
surgical removal of part of the cornea.

Lagophthalmos
inability to fully close the eyelids on blinking.

Lendectomy
surgical removal of the lens.

Lens luxation
dislocation of the lens from its normal position.

Limbus
the junction between the cornea and sclera.

Meibomian gland
gland within the eyelid margin producing lipid portion of tears.

Meibomianitis
inflammation of the meibomian glands.

Menace response
blinking of a patient when stimulated with a threatening gesture.

Microphakia
abnormally small lens.

Microphthalmos
abnormally small eye.

Miosis
constricted pupil.

Mydriasis
dilated pupil.

Myopia
short-sightedness.

Nasolacrimal punctae
drainage holes located close to medial canthus to drain tears.

Nuclear sclerosis
age-related hardening of the lens.

Neuro-ophthalmology
study of the cranial nerves and neurological aspects of ophthalmology.

Nyctalopia
night blindness.

Ophthalmoscopy
examination of the eye.

Ophthalmia neonatorum
conjunctivitis in newborn animal.

Optic nerve
cranial nerve II, carries visual impulses from the retina to the brain.

Optic disc
visible portion of the optic nerve in the fundus.

Optic neuritis
inflammation of the optic nerve.

Orbit
the bony surround to the eyeball and its contents.

Palpebral fissure
eyelid opening.

Pannus
superficial corneal vascularisation and granulation tissue.

Panophthalmitis
inflammation of all the ocular tissues.

Panuveitis
uveitis affecting the iris, choroid and ciliary body.

Papilloedema
swelling (oedema) of the optic disc.

Paracentesis
sample collection from the anterior chamber.

Pectinate ligaments
structures crossing the iridocorneal angle through which aqueous drains.

Phacoemulsification
technique for cataract extraction.

Photophobia
sensitivity to light.

Photoreceptor
light sensitive cell in the retina.

Phthisis bulbi
pathological shrinkage of the globe.

Posterior chamber
posterior part of the anterior segment between the iris and lens.

Posterior segment
posterior section of the globe between the lens and retina (filled with vitreous).

Progressive retinal atrophy
progressive degeneration of the retina, often inherited.

Proptosis
forward displacement of the globe.

Pupil
hole in the centre of the iris through which light passes.

Pupillary membrane
vascular membrane over the iris which normally regresses, but can be retained as persistent pupillary membrane (PPM) remnants.

Retina
innermost, light sensitive layer of the back of the eye.

Retinal dysplasia
abnormal differentiation of the retinal layers.

Retinal pigment epithelium (RPE)
metabolically active layer of the retina.

Retinopathy
disease of the retina (e.g. hypertensive retinopathy).

Retrobulbar space
area between the sclera and the back of the orbit.

Rhodopsin
photoreceptor pigment found in rods.

Rhytidectomy
face-lift procedure.

Rod
photoreceptor cell sensitive in low light levels.

Rubeosis iridis
increased vascularisation of the iris, usually with inflammation.

Schirmer tear test reading
measurement of aqueous tear production.

Sclera
outer fibrous coat of the eye normally white in colour.

Sequestrum (corneal)
feline corneal disease characterised by darkly pigmented plaque and ulceration.

Stades procedure
surgery for upper lid entropion/trichiasis resulting in forced granulation at the eyelid margin.

Strabismus
squint.

Stye
inflammation of an eyelid gland.

Subluxation
partial displacement of the lens.

Symblepharon
abnormal conjunctival adhesions.

Synchisis scintillans
presence of cholesterol crystals in liquefied vitreous.

Synechia
adhesions of the iris (anterior to cornea, posterior to lens).

Syneresis
vitreal liquefaction.

Tapetum
the reflective layer in the dorsal choroid (also called tapetum lucidum).

Tarsorrhaphy
surgical closure of the eyelids (temporary or permanent).

Tarsal plate
the supporting layer of the eyelid.

Tissue plasminogen activator (tPA)
substance used to lyse blood and fibrin clots.

Tonometry
measurement of intraocular pressure.

Trichiasis
ocular irritation caused by hairs in their normal position rubbing on the eye, e.g. from nasal folds.

Uvea/uveal tract
the vascular, often pigmented, layer of the globe consisting of iris, ciliary body and choroid.

Uveitis
inflammation of the uveal tract.

Viscoelastic
thick gel used during intraocular surgery.

Vitrectomy
surgical removal of the vitreous.

Vitreous
the hydro-gel filling the posterior segment.

Vitreocentesis
collection of samples from the vitreous for laboratory analysis.

Zonules
supporting fibres of the lens attached to the ciliary body.

Index

Page numbers in **bold** indicate figures and tables; *a* denotes appendix; *g* refers to glossary.